What is Your
Nutritional Deficiency?

Find it, Fix it, and Feel Better!

Also by Dr. Howard F. Loomis, Jr.

Enzymes: The Key to Health, Volume 1,
The Fundamentals

The Enzyme Advantage: For Health Care Providers
and People Who Care About Their Health

The Enzyme Advantage: For Women

What is Your Nutritional Deficiency?

Find it, Fix it, and Feel Better!

Howard F. Loomis, Jr.

D.C., F.I.A.C.A.

with Arnold Mann

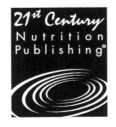

Cover design, layout: Camron Lewis
Editor: Meredith H. Pond

Library of Congress Cataloging-in-Publication Data
Loomis, Howard F.
What is Your Nutritional Deficiency?
Find it, Fix it, and Feel Better!
Includes references and index.
1. Enzymes. 2. Nutrition. 3. Digestion. 4. Deficiency.
Mann, Arnold.

First Edition, Printed in the USA

ISBN 978-0-9769124-4-6

DISCLAIMER: This book is not about treating disease, and no information
contained in it should be construed as such. This book is about how plant
enzymes can be used to deliver nutrition, for the purpose of restoring
normal function and maintaining health. When making dietary changes,
please remember to consult your health care practitioner.

Dedication

"It is the mark of an educated mind to be able to entertain a thought without accepting it."
—Aristotle

"Howard, think, examine, and analyze. Don't just accept."
—Dr. Earl Lankau, Logan Chiropractic College, 1965

To Pamela Warner, Fran Anderson, and Cheryl Rupard, three educated and dedicated minds who patiently provided guidance and assistance in the development of my work.
Thank you.

Table of Contents

Foreword

By Dr. Ivan Kelley

As a fellow chiropractor and ardent follower of Dr. Howard Loomis' work for well over thirty years, I am exceedingly honored to have the opportunity to share why this book can and will be of such importance to you and your loved ones.

I first met Dr. Loomis in 1985 at a meeting with the owners of Rainbow Light Nutritional Systems in Santa Cruz, California. Fifteen minutes into the meeting, I was spell-bound. These were not the types of enzymes I expected. Somehow, none of the classes in any of my schools or programs – two bachelor of science degrees, a masters degree, Doctor of Chiropractic, certified nutritional consultant, certified clinical nutritionist, a diplomate of the American Chiropractic Board of Nutrition – addressed the existence or importance of food enzymes.

This meeting changed my professional life. Up to this point, my successes with nutritional consulting had been hit or miss at best. After hearing of Dr. Loomis' personal study with Dr. Edward Howell, I began reading everything I could find about food enzymes and, more specifically, supplemental predigestive enzymes.

A tremendous amount has been written since Dr. Howell's short manuscript in 1934 entitled *"Are Food Enzymes Important in Digestion and Metabolism?"* He then published *The Status of Food Enzymes in Digestion and Metabolism* in 1946. It was reprinted as *Food Enzymes for Health & Longevity* in 1980. His final book, *Enzyme Nutrition, the Food Enzyme Concept*, was published in 1985. Numerous rereadings always provide new insights.

In 1999, Dr. Loomis began presenting seminars to train health care professionals in his techniques for evaluating patients to determine the unique areas of stress causing their health problems. This involved an in-depth history, laboratory work (blood tests and 24-hour urinalysis) and a detailed physical examination. With this information, a practitioner could confidently advise a patient/client about dietary changes and specific food enzyme formulas created by Dr. Loomis. Years of testing (often on himself) refined his formulas, and added new ones, so anyone recommending them could be confident they would see changes with re-evaluations. Hit and miss nutritional work became a thing of the past.

At the beginning of the first several annual training seminars, Dr. Loomis would have someone from the hotel staff bring him a glass bowl of very thick, warm oatmeal. Like a magician, he would take a capsule from a bottle of enzymes, open it, and sprinkle the powdered contents on the oatmeal before returning the bowl to the front of the class. Shortly, someone would either notice and mention the oatmeal changing or Dr. Loomis would pick up the bowl again. Much to the amazement of the audience, the thick oatmeal would now be a thin, runny, almost clear liquid. This was always an effective segue to his explanations for why supplemental enzymes were essential for human digestion.

One of the best parts of these seminars was relearning things we all should have known from school in new, creative ways. Dr. Loomis' quiet, gentle delivery and depth of knowledge allowed everyone to comprehend previously misunderstood or poorly-learned concepts. His mastery of physiology, along with his ability to clearly and concisely explain how and why things worked, was the primary reason I frequently recommended Dr. Loomis' training to other health care professionals. I always said, "You'll learn and understand biochemistry like never before." The consensus was one hundred percent agreement.

Putting this knowledge to work clinically provides consistent results. The joy of helping people overcome health issues and improve their lives never diminishes. It's the primary reason I have no plans, after 34 years, of retiring any time soon.

Personally experiencing the results of this treatment program is something else entirely.

Briefly summarized, in 2009 I learned to truly appreciate the unrelenting agony and disability of low back and leg pain from a MRI-confirmed ruptured lumbar disc. I declined the recommended surgery. Prescriptive pain pills and muscle relaxers proved useless. After several sleepless nights (we are always our own worst patients), I began taking very high doses of two of Dr. Loomis' enzyme formulas every waking hour. I slept that night. Within a week, I was back at work part time. Within six months, I was walking without limping. I remain fully functional.

I'm pretty sure I've read every article and book Dr. Loomis has written. What has remained fascinating and amazing is how his teachings have never deviated from Dr. Howell's original concepts. Today, their roles are somewhat reversed. Dr. Howell formed the National Enzyme Company (NEC) in 1932 to promote his enzyme formulas for pre-digestion. Mr. Tony Collier took over NEC in 1978. This small mail-order firm finally became a hugely successful, worldwide operation after Dr. Loomis began working with Tony to develop formulas and train healthcare providers. In 1993, Dr. Loomis formed Enzyme Formulations to produce his own formulas.

With this book, Dr. Loomis returns to the importance of Dr. Howell's original concept. Naturally occurring enzymes in raw foods are destroyed to extend shelf life. Depleted soils, and many other factors, diminish the nutrient value of today's raw foods. With fewer food enzymes available, our bodies must use more of their own enzyme reserves to complete digestion. This escalating enzyme deficiency frequently manifests as problems digesting one or more of our primary sources of energy – carbohydrates, proteins, or fats. Without the energy/ the fuel to repair and replace as well as to maintain normal immune function, our overall health suffers. Neither vitamins, minerals, man-made supplements, nor drugs can provide energy or replace depleted enzymes.

Enjoy reading as Dr. Loomis helps you discover *What's Your Nutritional Deficiency?*

Introduction

Twenty years ago, I wrote a book called *Enzymes: The Key to Health*, in which I extolled the virtues of naturally occurring enzymes, especially those found in fruits and vegetables. At the time, nutritional experts were recommending that we consume five to nine servings of fresh fruits and vegetables every day to maintain our health.

That recommendation stands today, though it has nothing to do with enzymes. It does not account for the fact that the enzymes Nature placed in those fruits and vegetables to facilitate the ripening process also assist our body's own digestive enzymes. These enzymes predigest the foods they occur in naturally, helping us absorb and use the vital nutrients they provide.

Few nutritional experts are aware of the key predigestive role these food enzymes play in the human body, and the fact that today's produce is not what it used to be. Out of necessity, the food industry—via chemical treatment and genetic modification—has all but eliminated Nature's enzymes from today's produce. Why? To achieve increased shelf life. So, the concept of eating fresh fruits and vegetables to maintain health is not as valid as it once was. Food enzymes from other sources, such as meats, grains and dairy products, were killed off long ago, as they continue to be, by cooking, processing and pasteurization.

The price we pay for the loss of these essential nutrients is twofold. First, there's the extra workload placed on the body to produce enough enzymes over a lifetime to digest and assimilate all the foods we consume. Second, there are the consequences of our declining ability to do so on our overall health and well-being, especially regarding our increased risk of developing chronic degenerative diseases, such as arthritis and heart disease.

What is being promoted today for maintaining health is a vast array of pharmaceutical-grade vitamin and mineral supplements. My own first encounter with these supplements came in 1954. I was a junior in high school, and my mother, who had been trained as a nurse, took me with her to the drug store. I stood beside her as she surveyed the shelves. I remember seeing all the vitamin and mineral preparations and thinking, my God, how confusing is this!

"What are you looking for?" I asked her, and she said thoughtfully, "Well, I'm not quite certain just yet."

My brother had just broken his arm. My father had suffered a severe lower back injury in an automobile accident. He had sold his business and enrolled in a chiropractic college. Mother was working full time at an office job. These were stressful times for our family, and we were all feeling a bit fatigued.

So, what should she buy?

I remember her picking up various bottles of vitamin A and vitamin D and looking at the labels. In 1954, vitamins and minerals were just beginning to be marketed. Vitamin C wasn't even discovered until 1928, let alone manufactured. Most of this stuff came out after World War II. My parents were part of that generation; so, this was all relatively new to them.

Finally, her eye caught sight of the only thing on the shelves that made any sense to her—a bottle of cod liver oil. As a nurse trained in the 1930s, she knew what cod liver oil was used for. In her day, it had been shown to prevent rickets and other symptoms of vitamin D deficiency. She knew cod liver oil had high levels of vitamin D in it, as well as vitamin A. Symptoms of a vitamin D deficiency include muscle weakness, bone pain, fractures and unexplained fatigue. The cod liver oil came from a natural source, as opposed to a concentrated, isolated pharmaceutical-grade vitamin. She knew she could give us cod liver oil between meals and our bodies would absorb and use it. She'd seen its good results for years.

The confusion over vitamin and mineral supplements continues to this day, in large part because the symptoms of their deficiencies overlap so much. Scurvy, the end result of a vitamin C deficiency, was once a scourge among sailors who endured for months at sea without so much as a piece of citrus fruit or even a tomato. Then doctors figured out what caused it. Scurvy is rarely seen today, except in developing nations, or in areas where severe malnutrition occurs.

And yet, if viewed as a disease process, the early signs of scurvy are quite common.

Vitamin C deficiency produces scurvy in 60 to 90 days. However, the early symptoms of the deficiency include weakness and feeling tired all the time. The person can become irritable. Gradually, the joints in the arms and legs begin to stiffen. Then the person's joints begin to hurt, followed by small bruises appearing on their arms and legs for no apparent reason.

These are the earliest signs of a vitamin C deficiency. Without treatment, the person will soon notice pink on their toothbrush, as they develop gum disease and their teeth start to loosen. Bleeding from the skin may also occur. All of this can lead to poor wound healing, and finally death from infection or bleeding.

If a person shows up with full-blown scurvy, the doctor will know what to give them. But when viewed as a nutritional process, its early symptoms are very similar to those seen in a dozen other vitamin and mineral deficiencies.

As always, the key is to stop the progression before it reaches the disease state. Unfortunately, pharmaceutical vitamin supplements are not the answer. Recent studies have demonstrated that these supplements are not effective in reducing one's risk of developing the chronic degenerative diseases they are being marketed to prevent. This makes sense, because vitamins and minerals don't have the capacity to perform any work. They have to be put to work by enzymes—*if* they get absorbed at all. It's been said that the American people have the most expensive urine in the world.

Total vitamin deficiencies are rarely seen today. If anything, the American public is guilty of overeating. So, it's not a deficiency of vitamins and minerals we should be concerned about. The key to staying healthy, besides eating the right foods, is maintaining our ability to digest and use the nutrients good foods contain, and not exhausting our body's ability to produce enzymes to do this over time.

It's All About Energy

The body needs energy to keep all its organ systems running in homeostatic harmony. Its three sources of energy are carbohydrates, proteins and lipids (fats). The body's preferred source for energy is carbohydrates—complex carbohydrates such as in vegetables, not refined sugars. When the body runs out of carbohydrates, it turns to protein for energy. Amino acids, which are normally used for growth and repair, are removed from body cells and sent to the liver for conversion to glucose. When that source runs low, lipids are pulled out of storage and sent to the liver, which begins converting them to glucose for energy. This results in the elevation of triglycerides and glucose in the blood, which can lead to metabolic syndrome and Type II diabetes. The entire process of finding alternative sources of energy, when long continued, can be said to be the beginning of chronic illnesses.

The key to relieving symptoms and halting the progression to illness and degeneration is figuring out what the nutritional deficiency is when symptoms first appear, and then giving the body the nutrition/energy it needs to get the struggling organ system or systems back on track and running properly. Sounds simple but . . . It's not just about consuming the right nutrients; it's about getting these nutrients absorbed into the body.

According to the Council on Nutrition of the American Medical Association, nutrition is "the science of food: what is ingested, digested, absorbed, transported, utilized, and eliminated." According to *Dorland's Medical Dictionary*, food is "anything which, when taken into the body, serves to nourish or build up the tissues or to supply body heat," or the energy that comes from breaking down and using the available nutrients. Of course, the breaking-down process itself also requires energy.

Once again, it all comes down to enzymes.

Without adequate digestive enzymes from saliva and the pancreas to do the digestive work—amylase to digest carbohydrates, protease to digest proteins, and lipase to digest fats—the nutrients we consume will never enter the body. In other words, if they are not broken down to an absorbable state, they will never cross the intestinal wall and be used for energy.

Furthermore, these essential compounds—enzymes—are also used to create other equally essential compounds. For example, protein is used to create insulin, thyroxine, hemoglobin, epinephrine, neurotransmitters and dopamine-serotonin. Lipids are broken down to fatty acids, prostaglandins, phospholipids, sterols, cholesterol and sex hormones.

Are you having any reproductive issues? Reproductive hormones are all derived from lipids.

The Mood Cascade

One of the most common features of a nutritional deficiency is the **mood cascade** that occurs as our body goes from burning carbohydrates to proteins to lipids for energy.

When someone becomes protein deficient, they start losing calcium into their urine, because it is protein that binds to and transports calcium in the blood. Hence, the person becomes a little irritable, which is a symptom of calcium deficiency. But it's really the protein deficiency—not enough protein in the diet, a failure to digest the protein, or burning protein for energy—that's the source of the problem.

A lipid deficiency can be due to inadequate stomach acid, which stimulates the flow of bile, which emulsifies lipids so that the digestive enzymes can penetrate them. The lipid-deficient person can become choleric, or crabby and testy, or even downright cantankerous!

The person who is becoming carbohydrate deficient will first move into a state of melancholy. When they turn to simple sugars as a source of energy, they experience a depletion of alkaline minerals. So, they go for the quick energy fix from the sugar hit, which is followed by the inevitable collapse—and they become apathetic, uninterested and detached from the life around them.

It's all about looking at the symptoms and asking the question: What is my deficiency? In determining the answer, we are looking at either inadequate ingestion or digestion of essential nutrients. You can eat a ton of protein, but if you don't have the enzymes to digest it, it will never be absorbed into your body and you will be protein deficient.

Or if you are under stress and your body runs out of carbohydrates and starts burning protein for energy, you can become protein deficient.

No matter how you look at it, your enzymes are the key to digesting, absorbing and using the nutrients from the foods you eat.

About this Book

The purpose of this book is to look at what you may be doing to exhaust your enzyme potential—your body's ability to produce the digestive enzymes and the metabolic enzymes that are the life force behind every biochemical process taking place in every organ and every biological nook and cranny of your body.

Chapter by chapter, we will look at how the human body uses its own enzymes to digest the food we take in, how we can easily exhaust them trying to compensate for the enzymes which are no longer in our food, and how the declining ability to do so as we age can put us on the road toward chronic degenerative diseases.

The science of nutrition, as explained by the American Medical Association, is the science of food, not the science of vitamins and minerals. It's about what is ingested, digested, absorbed, transported, used and eliminated. All of this is driven by the enzyme systems in your body.

My goal in writing this book is to enable you to see why you are energy deficient—why you are fatigued, why you are apathetic, and why a host of other symptoms may appear as your organs struggle to perform under an energy shortage. We're going to trace that energy shortage back to food, and how vitamins and minerals are used by enzymes in your body to produce essential compounds. Those essential compounds hold the secret to preventing chronic degenerative diseases.

The pages that follow will serve as a guide for you to understand how your body is struggling to produce energy and how your symptoms can be relieved by providing the nutrition your body needs.

— Dr. Howard F. Loomis, Jr.
Madison, Wisconsin, 2019

Chapter 1

It's All About Energy!

The most common symptom complained of in a doctor's office is fatigue, or lack of energy. It is fair to say fatigue underlies every nutritional problem. This book is about energy—how the body gets energy, how the body uses energy, how to recognize an energy deficiency, and how daily occurring symptoms can tell us what the body needs nutritionally to get it back on course before it reaches a "disease state."

> **The human body must produce energy for three distinct purposes:**
> 1. For the brain to maintain cognitive and emotional stability, and to drive all body systems.
> 2. For the musculoskeletal system to oppose gravity and facilitate movement.
> 3. To transport and supply nutrients to all body cells, tissues and organs so they can function in harmony.

When one or more of these systems become deficient because of overwork, or due to a lack of nutrients, symptoms result.

It's all about energy.

The human body has three sources of energy— carbohydrates, protein and fat, all of which must be converted to glucose to be used as fuel. In times of stress, the body will save its glucose for the brain and instruct other cells to burn fat.

The body prefers carbohydrates as its primary source of energy because it's a high-energy food easily converted into energy by the cells. However, carbohydrates are not stored widely in the body—only in the liver and the muscles, as an emergency source of energy. While muscles store glucose, in the form of glycogen, this glucose can only be used by the muscles in the event of a "fight or flight" situation.

When the body does not have enough carbohydrates, it turns to protein. Each cell hoards protein in the form of amino acids, which it can use to repair itself or to reproduce. When the carbohydrate supply is exhausted and an alternate source of energy is needed, the brain instructs cells to send their amino acids to the liver to be converted to glucose. This means that anybody who is under stress for any length of time— be it biochemical, structural or emotional stress—is going to become protein deficient.

Only when the body is protein deficient will it turn to lipids, or fats, for energy.

While every cell in the body can use fat for energy if the need arises, the brain is not able to convert fat to glucose fast enough to keep working efficiently. It needs high-octane fuel. The brain gets first dibs on all available glucose, from the moment it senses the first sweet drop being digested by salivary amylase at work in the mouth, to the craving that comes when glucose is not present.

It's all about energy, and the body's ability to digest what it takes in. Or the body's failure to do so and the consequences. As this chapter continues, you will see how it can be a struggle for a body to get the energy it needs.

Pitfalls of Clinical Specialization

If there is one thing in medicine today that often works against our overall health and well-being, it is the fact that the study of the human body has been divided conceptually into its different organ systems—respiratory, circulatory, musculoskeletal, urinary and reproductive, for example. This has resulted in clinical specialization along these lines within the various healing arts. As useful as this systemic approach may have been since the advent of specialized medicine, it has also meant that coordination between existing professions and specialties has become very difficult when it comes to diagnosis and treatment.

Take, for example, the Digestive System.

It might come as a complete surprise, but there is no clinical specialty that emphasizes restoring normal digestion, or normal digestive function. Perhaps this is because symptoms emanating from the stomach, the gallbladder, the pancreas or the small intestine, are very difficult to identify until a person has reached a state of full-blown disease. Hence, early warning signs often escape clinical detection because it's hard to tell where the symptoms are coming from.

For this reason, the use of antacids, proton pump inhibitors and H2 blockers to neutralize or block stomach acid from forming as a means of relieving symptoms has become common. When needed, a prescription is readily available, or they may simply be purchased over-the-counter.

What is not commonly understood by patients is that many pharmaceutical drugs, including over-the-counter remedies, are designed to interfere with or block a normal enzyme-driven physiological function. This approach relieves symptoms and presumably will prevent a disease process from developing. However, all drugs also have side effects, precisely because they are designed to block normal body functions. The pharmaceutical approach is necessary to treat a disease process, but it is not designed to restore normal function.

For example, using a proton pump inhibitor to shut down stomach acid production and relieve heartburn also impairs protein digestion, as well as bile flow, which in turn impairs fat digestion.

And so, relief of symptoms comes at a cost, especially when the symptoms reappear frequently and use of the medication may eventually result in a chronic degenerative process other than the one it was intended to prevent. Recent studies have shown that long-term use of acid-blocking drugs can cause spontaneous fractures and sudden onset of kidney failure.

The more prudent approach to relieving symptoms, when a specific disease process cannot be identified, would be to identify the source of the symptoms and then give the body the specific nutrition it needs to restore normal function to a struggling organ or organ system, thus maintaining health and preventing disease.

Key to this approach is the body's ability to digest, absorb and use the nutrition it is receiving.

This is where predigestion comes in.

Digestion officially begins in the stomach with the formation of stomach acid, or hydrochloric acid, which converts pepsinogen into protein-digesting pepsin. That's the official take. And yet, it takes 45 minutes after we begin eating before hydrochloric acid forms in the stomach.

This is in young, healthy adults. As we age, it can take much longer than 45 minutes.

> To relieve digestive symptoms by restoring normal digestive function, we must first recognize and understand the essential role of "predigestion," which begins the moment food enters the mouth, and which does not receive the respect it deserves in the health sciences.

Presumptions of Fact

The reason that predigestion is not widely recognized has to do with the presumption of "scientific fact," which can (and often does) get in the way of true understanding and scientific progress. This phenomenon is eloquently described by Dr. Lisa Rosenbaum in her May 2017 *New England Journal of Medicine* essay entitled, "The March of Science—The True Story."

Dr. Rosenbaum's opening quote, from the 17th century's Father of Empiricism, Sir Francis Bacon, says it all: "The human understanding when it has once adopted an option ... draws all things else to support and agree with it."

In other words, once we decide that something is true, we close our minds to opposing opinions and seek to justify our beliefs, even if they are not well-founded.

Taking it one step further, Rosenbaum quotes Harvard psychologist Daniel Gilbert, who recalls "the warning many of us hear on the first day of medical school: 'Half of what we're going to teach you is wrong—the problem is, we don't know which half.' "

Then there are those great iconoclastic moments that change our thinking altogether. Until Australian physician Barry Marshall drank a petri dish full of H-pylori bacteria, which he had collected from his patients' stomachs, the medical world mocked him for even suggesting that bacteria might be in any way associated with gastritis or peptic ulcer disease. Bacteria can't survive in the acid stomach. Everybody knew that.

The international ridicule continued, until Marshall cured himself and many of his patients with a course of antibiotics.

Marshall was eventually awarded the Nobel Prize for his discovery, and for helping to bring an epidemic under control.

His work also reveals that using acid-blocking drugs long term can put a person at risk for a bacterial overgrowth in the stomach lining because bacteria flourish in an alkaline (non-acidic) environment.

This brings us to predigestion.

The misconception holding back recognition of predigestion also has to do with stomach acid.

> It is an assumed "scientific certainty" within the medical community that predigestion does not occur in the human body because stomach acid would destroy any digestive enzymes before they have a chance to go to work.

This "certainty" is stated by many "experts" in their writings and online pontifications—even though all basic physiology textbooks clearly state otherwise.

A case in point is a reader comment made about Dr. Louis De Palma's 2007 book, *You Take Too-Big-A Bite!* The story takes children on a fun journey through their own digestive tracts, extolling the values of taking the time to eat the proper foods and to chew foods thoroughly. The reviewer, who identifies herself as a college teacher of physiology and chemistry, declares Dr. De Palma to be "flat wrong" in his assertion that enzymes contained in the raw fruits and vegetables we consume play any role in digestion. Why? Because, she insists, the enzymes are made of protein and just like any other proteins, they would be broken down in our "very acidic" stomach.

It follows that any digestive enzymes produced by the salivary glands would also be destroyed by stomach acid before they have a chance to do any work.

In fact, all the above is "flat wrong," because, as noted, it takes the body at least 45 minutes to produce stomach acid once we begin a meal. Prior to this, any enzymes contained in our saliva, or in the foods we consume, would play an important role in our predigestion of these foods.

While it is not generally taught in nutrition classes, it is well documented in all the physiology books that salivary enzymes continue to work in the stomach until hydrochloric acid is formed, creating an acid environment in which those enzymes can no longer work.

This is not a new concept, it has been known for over 100 years. Allow me to quote from *The Mechanical Factors of Digestion* written by Walter B. Cannon in 1911. (Cannon is regarded as the Father of Modern Physiology). "As long ago as 1880, Von den Velden pointed out that free hydrochloric acid does not appear for almost an hour after eating an ordinary breakfast, and for almost 2 hours after eating a full midday meal." Make no mistake, while research and technology have advanced greatly since then, body functions have not!

But up to that point, prior to the formation of stomach acid, studies have shown that salivary enzymes alone can predigest 50 percent of starch (within the first 15 minutes!), up to 30 percent of protein and up to 10 percent of fat.

This is a major contributing factor to our body's ability to digest and assimilate the nutrients we consume to maintain normal function and healthy well-being.

Let's take a closer look at predigestion Nature's way.

Digestion Begins in the Mouth

The digestive process begins with chewing, where large food particles are broken up into smaller particles. The importance of this initial stage of digestion is often overlooked. Not only is chewing needed so food can be swallowed without choking, it is also necessary to expose as much surface area to the food particles as possible so the enzymes can penetrate them and begin digestion.

Next, the salivary glands go to work secreting mucus into the mouth, which combines with water to moisten and lubricate the food particles prior to swallowing. Besides facilitating swallowing, this lubrication of food also protects the mucosal surfaces of the mouth, throat and the esophagus from irritation as the food moves along the downward pathway to the stomach.

Besides water and mucus, saliva also contains digestive enzymes: amylase, protease and lipase, which are essential for initiating predigestion in the mouth and the stomach.

Amylase is secreted from the parotid glands, which are located near the ears, and breaks down carbohydrates/starches into smaller molecules.

Protease is secreted from the submandibular glands, located in the region of the lower jaw, and can initiate protein digestion. My college biochemistry textbook from the 1960s stated that this was a safeguard against bacteria. Certainly, much more is known today about the presence of protease in the saliva.

Lipase is secreted from the sublingual glands, located under the tongue, to initiate fat digestion. Due to its unique characteristics, its activity continues in the stomach, even in the presence of stomach acid. As much as 30 percent of fat is digested within 1 to 20 minutes of ingestion by lingual lipase alone.

It is often forgotten that the natural enzymes contained in the foods that we consume—if they are still intact— also begin working in the mouth. One of these enzymes, cellulase, is not made by the human body. Our only source of cellulase is fibrous fruits and vegetables that contain it. Nutrition books seldom talk about this. They simply recommend a high-fiber diet.

Cellulase digests soluble fiber, as opposed to insoluble fiber which cannot be digested. This is of critical importance because the vegetables that contain cellulase are covered with a thin coating of cellulose. If that cellulose is not removed by cooking, it must be chewed off, because human enzymes cannot penetrate that protective layer. If it is not cooked, or if the fruit or vegetable is not fully chewed, the person will develop gas when eating raw food.

And so, we arrive at a contradiction in nutritional terms.

While we are encouraged to eat fresh fruits and vegetables to stay healthy, cooking is often promoted as a "digestive aide." That's the way it appears in nutrition books. No reference is made to the predigestive role played by the natural food enzymes in fruits and vegetables, or the fact that cooking destroys their ability to fulfill that role. Nor is there mention of the removal of these food enzymes to achieve increased shelf life. The advice is simply to cook the cellulose off one's fruits and vegetables to better digest them.

What is the point of eating fresh fruits and vegetables if we are unable to sufficiently digest them?

When I was in practice, I kept noticing that the sickest people I saw ate the best diet. They were eating a high-fiber diet of fresh fruits and vegetables in which the natural enzymes had been removed, and they weren't cooking what they ate. So, they couldn't adequately digest it.

If, on the other hand, the fibrous fruits and vegetables we consume still contain the enzymes Nature put in them, all we need do is chew thoroughly to break the food apart, release the enzymes—cellulase included—and get the full benefit of the nutrients therein.

Such is Nature's design.

In Nature's design, chewing remains essential to good overall digestion and assimilation of nutrients contained in fresh fruits and vegetables, as well as other foods we consume.

Besides enzymes, the saliva our body creates also contains an assortment of minerals. These mineral ions, which include sodium, potassium, magnesium, calcium, chloride, bicarbonate phosphate and iodine, activate chemical receptors in the mouth, giving rise to the sensation of taste. Reduced water content and an imbalance of minerals can cause a metallic taste in the mouth.

These minerals also maintain the pH within the mouth, keeping the acidity within a certain range—typically slightly acid or slightly alkaline. This helps prevent deterioration of tooth enamel.

The mineral content of saliva is critical. It is under the direct control of the central nervous system. Both the sympathetic and the parasympathetic branches work to control the concentration of the alkaline and acid elements of saliva.

It is the sympathetic system that responds to stress—not just emotional stress, but also stress from a visceral organ system that is not performing adequately and is producing symptoms, and even when there is a structural stress or injury. Under such stress, besides having specific effects on the heart and the lungs, as well as the muscles, the sympathetic nervous system also reduces digestive activity and movement of food throughout the digestive tract. It also reduces the amount of water in the saliva, which compromises the taste buds and the action of its digestive enzyme secretion.

Hence, predigestion is impaired when one is under chronic stress—be it structural, biochemical or emotional stress.

Finally, while we don't usually think about saliva having a bactericidal effect, when consistently low levels are secreted, the risk of dental cavities and even fungal infections, such as oral candidiasis, are increased.

So, one could say that the function of saliva and its mineral content is to maintain good oral hygiene for the predigestion of foods in the "predigestive" stomach, before stomach acid takes over.

It's all part of Nature's plan.

And now, we head into the stomach.

Gastric Digestion

The stomach is flat when empty. It begins to stretch when food enters the upper part, or the fundus. As more food arrives, the stomach wall stretches accordingly. It is this stretching that signals the body to begin the complicated process of forming hydrochloric acid. As noted, it takes 45 minutes for the stomach acid to form and begin doing its work, converting pepsinogen into pepsin to digest protein. Again, this is in young, healthy adults. People past the age of 40 generally require a longer time, and most of those entering their Social Security years are unable to concentrate enough stomach aid to initiate protein digestion adequately.

Many of Nature's creatures—grazing animals in particular—have an extra stomach, or chamber, where the enzymes contained in the foods being eaten begin digesting these foods. Humans do not have an extra stomach per se, but this upper cardiac portion of the human stomach is analogous in function, serving as the predigestive chamber until the hydrochloric acid forms in the expanding middle portion of the stomach.

During this waiting period, the salivary enzymes and any enzymes contained in the ingested food continue the process begun in the mouth. Studies indicate that at least 40 to 80 percent of starches (complex carbohydrates) can be digested within 15 minutes, with averages running at 60 percent of starches, 30 percent of protein and 10 percent of fat.

All this occurs before the stomach begins its own digestion.

The brain knows exactly what it's doing when it comes to formulating saliva content because that 60/30/10 ratio with regards to carbohydrate, protein and fat predigestion respectively is precisely what is needed to accommodate the way the body uses each of these nutritional elements for energy.

The whole purpose of predigestion is to deliver energy to the body as soon as possible.

If you can start digesting carbohydrates—the body's preferred energy source—before hydrochloric acid starts protein digestion, the body will take it in.

This was observed in a University of Toronto study back in the 1950s. The researchers wanted to know where glucose is absorbed in the body. They attached a radioisotope to the glucose molecules so they could follow them with a Geiger Counter-type instrument as the molecules made their way through the body. As it turned out, the study was cancelled because in every single patient the glucose was absorbed out of the mouth and into the brain within 20 seconds.

The Bottom Line

Glucose is energy, and the brain is a glucose hog.

Enzymes and Essential Nutrients

This brings us back to the salivary enzyme cocktail prepared by the brain for predigestive purposes: amylase, protease and lipase, in that order, with amylase giving the brain the quick glucose hit it needs by going to work on carbohydrates right away, in the mouth.

The whole purpose of predigestion is to obtain energy quickly. If we start the digestive process before stomach acid begins digesting protein, the body will take these nutrients in.

Now isn't it odd that the number of macronutrients—carbohydrate, protein and lipids—that the body can predigest most quickly is in the same order in which the body produces energy on a cellular level, with the preferred energy source, carbohydrate, coming first, with up to 50 percent of starches digested in the predigestive stomach in the first 15 minutes?

When the body runs out of carbohydrate for energy, it is forced to pull protein in the form of stored amino acids from the cells and send them to the liver to be converted to glucose. And when that runs out, it pulls stored fat.

The same careful design applies to enzymes contained in the foods we eat.

When it comes to food enzymes, Nature has effectively put the exact amount in the enzyme mix to match the caloric amount of carbohydrate, protein and lipid in that food.

In other words, a food that is highest in carbohydrates is going to have more amylase than protease or lipase. A food that is high in protein is going to be high in protease. And a food that is high in fat, like bananas or olives, is going to have more lipase.

This is the way Nature set things up.

Unfortunately for us humans, the enzymes Nature put in the foods we eat are all but gone. What has not been cooked, processed and pasteurized out of existence is being sacrificed to facilitate increased shelf life, by chemical treatment and now genetic modification.

Fresh fruits and vegetables, which were our sole remaining source of natural food enzymes, are no longer what they used to be, enzymatically speaking.

This fact is having an impact on our ability to digest these foods and assimilate and use their nutrients. Further, the resulting extra work is being placed on our pancreatic enzymes which diminish as we age, and as the body works harder to produce the enzymes needed to provide the energy to keep all systems running in homeostatic harmony.

Our "enzyme potential" diminishes with age, as one pioneer in enzyme research, Dr. Edward Howell, once put it.

The Bottom Line

A failure to consume adequate nutrition or to adequately digest what we consume results in energy deficiencies, and deficiencies in the essential compounds derived from the macronutrients we ingest.

Common symptoms signaling when digestion is not up to par, or when a dietary modification is needed include the following:

- Stiff, sore joints
- Headache
- Heartburn
- Indigestion
- Gas pain/bloating
- Constipation and diarrhea
- Anxiety and irritability
- Restlessness and insomnia

The above symptoms are caused by energy deficiencies resulting in the diminished ability of a body system to meet the demands being placed upon it.

That's what this book is about.

The question is: Which macronutrient, or combination of macronutrients, is responsible for your symptoms of deficiency?

The Bottom Line

The whole point of this book is to explain the fact that if you are having problems digesting macronutrients— carbohydrates, proteins, lipids—you are going to develop deficiencies in the essential compounds that flow from those three macronutrients.

Those deficiencies are evidence of a chronic degenerative process going on in your body. It's not about vitamins and minerals. These and other nutritional supplements are merely building blocks, and must be broken down, reorganized, and delivered to the cells to be used within those cells to produce energy. And that takes energy.

Food enzymes are the only nutritional supplement that have the capacity to perform work. And that is the definition of energy. So, what's *your* deficiency?

Chapter 2

Managing Your Energy and Mood with Food

The title of this book—and the heart of this book—is *What is Your Deficiency?*

With that in mind, I have noted that symptoms **cannot** be resolved, either clinically or objectively, with vitamin and mineral supplements. While vitamins and minerals are important, they are minor players in the metabolism of the macronutrients in your diet. Together with the body's metabolic enzymes, vitamins and minerals are used to produce essential nutrients needed to maintain health.

This chapter is all about recognizing that fundamental truth of basic science.

Once again, it all comes down to the energy needed to maintain healthy normal functions.

To wit:

- Energy must be provided for your brain to maintain cognitive functions and emotional stability.

- That energy is also used to maintain normal functions in your major organs systems and other tissues.

- What is usually forgotten is that your body must have a continual source of energy to oppose gravity, regardless of the physical position you are in. That energy supply cannot and is not shared with the brain and other organs systems.

Without adequate energy for the above three areas, you will have symptoms of energy deficiency!

So, What is Your Deficiency? Let's Find Out!

Your body functions are arranged so that your brain will readily recognize any stimulus that challenges its need for energy in any of the above three functional areas. Your brain also knows how to make adequate energy for increased needs if it is given the ingredients (food) to convert to energy.

Consider the following:

Your Body's Preferences for Energy Production

1st Choice *CARBOHYDRATE*

Your body prefers carbohydrates from adequately digested fruits, vegetables and select grains.

2nd Choice *PROTEIN*

The cells in your body need amino acids for growth and repair, but cells can convert amino acids to energy in times of need.

Last Resort *LIPIDS*

The body stores lipids for conversion to energy in times of temporary crisis. But, serious health problems can begin to surface if this emergency source is continued for extended periods.

As previously mentioned, the body prefers carbohydrate as its main energy source—because fruits and vegetables, as well as some grains, are readily digestible. With salivary enzymes, these carbohydrate energy packages can even be absorbed into the body *before* stomach acid is made.

Tell-Tale Signs

What are the early warning signs that the body is struggling to maintain adequate energy from carbohydrates on a regular basis? The following symptoms come and go based on dietary intake—or lack thereof—and conversion to energy:

- Frequent periods of fatigue (lack of energy)
- Dry mouth, eyes, and nose ("I don't seem to be able to drink enough water; I am always thirsty.")
- Dry skin, which is usually attributed to lipid deficiency
- Occasional difficulty concentrating or maintaining focus
- Being easily startled ("jumping" when you are busy concentrating and someone speaks to you)

It is during these periods that the body is resorting to amino acids—the building blocks of proteins—stored in its cells as a temporary source of energy production. Instead of being used for growth and repair, these amino acids must be sent to the liver where they can be converted. Of course, that process itself takes energy. We are told that as much as 57 percent of our protein intake is often converted to energy. That's a lot of the body's protein consumption. We will be discussing this process at length in Chapter 4, as it relates to the typical symptoms of adult females who are protein deficient.

Fortunately, the body is not going to tear down its cells to continue furnishing its protein resources for energy production.

What early symptoms can we recognize that tell us the body has reached the point of protein deficiency? Four early symptoms include the following:

- Increased watery secretions in the mouth, nose and eyes—the opposite signs of carbohydrate deficiency (when everything starts to dry up)
- Water gain, swelling in the hands and feet
- Cold hands and feet
- Menstrual cramps, and leg cramps at night or when resting

These are the most common symptoms of protein deficiency. Unfortunately, these symptoms are often assigned to another cause by those who depend on blood tests to identify protein deficiency. The body must maintain adequate protein levels in the blood to sustain life. The amino acids I am referring to are taken from the cells.

Should you rush off and find a quick-fix remedy? No. Instead, just begin to recognize why these symptoms may be appearing for you. Paying attention to your body is important.

When the body reaches its limit for giving up the cellular protein-building blocks it would normally use for growth and repair, it turns to stored lipids (fat) as an alternative energy source. Now it is time to sit up, take notice, and begin to take remedial action.

The body is telling you that the physiological process it uses for short-term stressful emergencies—the physiological "fight or flight" cascade of events—is now being used *only* to produce energy. There are many more serious problems that can begin to occur if this situation continues. These possible problems will be discussed in Chapter 5. For now, let's recognize that lipids are used to make steroidal sex hormones (estrogen, progesterone, and testosterone to name three) and their production will become inadequate unless normal energy production in your body can be resumed.

What are the early warning signs that this scenario may be occurring? The major signs include:

- Dry skin

- Flaking and dandruff

- Too much hair in the hair brush

We will discuss more long-term effects of continued or chronic stress, often referred to as *metabolic syndrome,* in Chapter 5.

Now let's turn our attention back to the brain and its need for energy to maintain cognitive and emotional stability, remembering that the musculoskeletal system needs and maintains its own source of energy for use during movement, exercise, and for "fight or flight" survival emergencies.

The brain requires and consumes the most energy of all the organ systems, followed by the heart and the liver, in that order.

First and foremost, the brain's work is maintaining the functions needed to control and direct all body functions, including thoughts.

Emotional stress obviously comes into play here, but the brain will still direct whatever energy is needed to maintain all other body processes first and deal with emotional stress as best it can later. There have been some important research findings in the area concerning food and emotions. Let's start with the most recent and work our way backwards chronologically.

Diet and Depression

The role of diet in the development of depressive disorders and symptoms has become an important research focus over the past decade.

A habitually poor diet with increased consumption of "Western" processed foods has been shown to be associated with a greater likelihood of—or risk for—depression and anxiety.

In one study, researchers at Deakin University School of Medicine in Australia reviewed the data from 12 epidemiological studies looking at the possible relationship between an unhealthy diet and mental health in children and adolescents. What they found was "significant" evidence linking "unhealthy dietary patterns and poorer mental health." Further, the researchers observed "a consistent trend" for a good quality diet and better mental health.

These researchers concluded: "Findings highlight the potential importance of the relationship between dietary patterns or quality and mental health early in the life span."

Now for the adults.

Several observational studies have found an inverse association between adherence to a Mediterranean diet and the risk of depression.

In a study published in 2013, researchers in Spain at the University of Las Palmas found an inverse association between the low-fat Mediterranean diet and the risk of depression. The community-based study was designed to look at this healthy diet as a means of preventing cardiovascular disease in a population of men aged 55 to 80 and women aged 60 to 80 who were at high risk for cardiovascular disease. Of the men and women, 51 percent had Type II diabetes.

After 3 years, the Mediterranean diet supplemented with nuts had a beneficial effect on the risk of depression in patients with Type II diabetes.

Remember, as I noted, when the body uses lipids—i.e., fats— as an alternative energy source for any length of time, some "bad" things can happen. Well, here is a perfect example of how dietary changes can help. In Type II diabetes, not only are the blood levels of glucose high, but also lipids (triglycerides). The Mediterranean diet is high in good carbohydrates, which tend to lower triglycerides; thus, the body has a better source of energy, and this helps lower fat accumulation in the blood.

The Spanish researchers concluded: "The results suggest that a Mediterranean diet supplemented with nuts could exert a beneficial effect on the risk of depression" in patients with Type II diabetes.

So maybe your diet or what's missing from it or what you're not digesting deserves some attention.

Managing Your Mood with Food

In the late 1970s, scientists discovered that the brain produces three chemical messengers called neurotransmitters directly from the food we eat. Chemical messengers transmit signals along nerve fibers to body cells, which then respond to the message.

Two amino acids—tyrosine and tryptophan—are used to make the neurotransmitters that control your mood in the following ways:

- Dopamine and norepinephrine are alertness chemicals made specifically from the amino acid tyrosine.

- Serotonin is a calming chemical made from the amino acid tryptophan.

Almost all protein foods contain larger quantities of tyrosine than tryptophan. Therefore, eating protein alone provides plenty of tyrosine for alertness chemical production, and tryptophan for calming chemical production.

Now here's the catch:

- **If you eat protein alone,** and your brain is rapidly using dopamine and norepinephrine (during some activity), it will use tyrosine to produce more of these two neurotransmitters. This helps you be more alert and energetic.

- **If you eat carbohydrate alone** without protein, more tryptophan becomes available for your brain, and you will feel more relaxed, less anxious, and more focused.

You might be asking: If the neurotransmitters are made from amino acids, which are the building blocks of protein, how does eating carbohydrate alone help the body produce more calming chemicals from tryptophan? If you are interested in knowing the answer to this question, the chemistry is easy to understand.

Insulin is responsible for carrying glucose into cells for energy production. Insulin is also responsible for carrying amino acids (protein) into the brain. After a protein meal, since tyrosine is much more plentiful, any unused tryptophan continues to flow in the blood (attached to albumin). Then, when a high-carbohydrate meal is consumed, insulin is circulating in the blood, and tryptophan becomes available to be carried into the brain. This results in an increased amount of serotonin production that exerts a strong calming effect.

So, you can influence your brain and your emotional state with food—if you know the right foods to eat, and if you can digest them. We have yet another reason why it may not be such a good idea to turn off the first step in protein digestion by blocking stomach acid production.

Are You Sanguine, Choleric, Melancholy, or Apathetic?

Let's go back a little further in time, before the late 1970s, and visit some old terms that were used to describe a person's mood before we understood neurotransmitters. In fact, the following concepts have been around for thousands of years and are even found in the writings of some of the ancient healing systems such as Ayurveda from India, Traditional Chinese Medicine, and Unani Tibb from the Greek-Persian schools.

Symptom-free, normal physiological functions can only occur when adequate amounts of carbohydrate are available for energy production, and protein levels are adequate to maintain all its vital responsibilities, as well as to cover for any temporary energy shortfall.

Such fortunate individuals will maintain optimistic and positive attitudes, even in bad or difficult situations. They can be described as having a **SANGUINE DEMEANOR,** meaning they are hopeful, buoyant, confident, cheerful, and upbeat.

However, continued or prolonged structural, visceral, or emotional stress (the "fight or flight" response) increases blood flow to muscles and reduces blood flow to organs of digestion and elimination. This causes energy deficiencies.

The resulting inadequate stomach-acid production or insufficient dietary protein can lead to the following:

- Calcium deficiency and irritability

- Iron deficiency—poor oxygenation of tissues and energy deficiency

- Inadequate stomach acid, leading to reduced amounts of stomach acid entering the duodenum, causing thickening of bile and poor fat digestion, which leads to fatty-acid and fat-soluble vitamin deficiencies

These individuals gradually become short-tempered or irritable, and testy and cantankerous. They can be described as having a **CHOLERIC DEMEANOR.**

Poor fat metabolism leads to altered bowel movements, which are also caused by inadequate dietary fiber or inadequate chewing and digestion of starch and high-fiber foods.

Recall that complex carbohydrates are excellent sources of energy and provide alkaline minerals in combination with water-soluble (stress) vitamins. A deficiency of complex carbohydrates can lead to a **MELANCHOLY DEMEANOR** characterized by a sad or unhappy countenance. This type of individual is sometimes described as pensive, meaning they are withdrawn or engaged in deep or serious thought.

It is only natural that energy-deficient individuals will turn to simple carbohydrates or alcohol for a quick source of energy. Unfortunately, this depletes alkaline minerals and water-soluble vitamins and produces an **APATHETIC DEMEANOR.** This type of individual is best described as unemotional and stolid, showing no interest, and lacking in enthusiasm or concern. In extreme cases, these individuals can become placid and meek.

Ultimately, poor diet and inadequate digestion lead to what has been termed *metabolic syndrome.*

This is not a specific diagnosis but rather a combination of several disorders under one roof, so to speak, related to metabolism.

Metabolic syndrome is characterized by energy deficiency, poor fat digestion and excess consumption of a simple carbohydrate diet.

The syndrome culminates in a collection of diagnostic signs that often occur together, such as:

- Elevated blood pressure

- Elevated triglycerides

- Elevated fasting blood glucose

- High cholesterol with high LDLs and low HDL

That's quite a ride.

Now let's take a slightly easier method of understanding nutritional science and how we can come to grips with our symptoms and identify our real deficiency.

There is more information at the end of the book with further in depth physiology. See Reference Charts on pages 113-119.

Chapter 3

Carbohydrates

As we begin this chapter, let me say one thing, carbohydrates are a multi-faceted story. It's about fiber, it's about starch and it's about sugar, all of which play important roles in providing your body with the energy it needs to fuel its systems and maintain health, and affect the symptoms associated with a failure to do so. It's a fascinating story.

One cannot talk about carbohydrates without the low-carb diet coming to mind. Such was the case in February of 2000, when I was an invited speaker at a medical conference in Atlanta, Georgia. That very same week, low-carb diet gurus Robert Atkins and Barry Sears—each with their own spin on what had become a national weight loss craze—along with anti-low-carb guru Dean Ornish, were all participating in The USDA Great Nutrition Debate in Washington, D.C.

And so, during my talk, I pointed out what I regarded to be the elephant in the room at that highly touted and publicized debate, and which I predicted would be confirmed in the next day's papers—that none of the experts participating in that USDA-sponsored debate would say anything about digestion.

My prediction proved to be correct. How the body processes what it takes in and creates energy to sustain its life functions and the consequences of a failure to adequately do so—in a word, Digestion—was not discussed by any of the diet gurus in attendance.

·prises there.

had been severely attacked by the American Medical Association (AMA) when he published his first book introducing his revolutionary weight loss plan back in 1972. The whole idea behind the diet was to restrict carbohydrate intake to the point where the body would be forced to burn stored fat for energy. The AMA's concern: when the liver starts converting fat to glucose, ketones are formed. These highly acidifying chemicals wind up in the bloodstream. For a person with diabetes, too many ketones in the blood, the AMA feared, could cause that person's body to become way too acidic, to the point where the results could be life-threatening.

Atkins even had his dieters using test strips to monitor their urine for ketones to make sure their bodies were in fact burning fat, and they were losing weight.

The other thing that happens when the body starts burning stored fat for energy is that it loses water. The dramatic early weight loss Atkins dieters experience is somewhat due to water loss.

Further, by the time a person starts burning fat, they are protein deficient, because the body turns to protein for energy production before it starts pulling stored fat. As the person becomes protein deficient, they also become calcium deficient, because 50 percent of the calcium in our blood is bound to protein.

Someone who is protein and calcium deficient is going to have SYMPTOMS—anxiety, irritability, irregular sleep patterns, edema, lack of energy, fatigue, and so on.

I remember coming home to my practice from the Atlanta conference. Everyone was coming in with this wonderful new diet, and they were all constipated and had all the symptoms of calcium and protein deficiency.

Currently, the Atkins diet, which is still being sold under that name, has been substantially modified from the original concept.

The problem with all fad diets is that none of them work long term.

The Bottom Line

The body has its own healthful mechanisms. If you feed it properly, giving it the nutrition it needs, if you get adequate rest, enough water and adequate exercise, the body will be likely to maintain normal function without symptoms.

If you want to lose weight, the best way to do it is simply cut down on calories and start to exercise.

It's not a good idea to deprive the body of its primary source of energy. That's the way Nature set things up, with carbohydrates first—complex carbohydrates—protein second, and fat as the last resort for energy.

Again, it's all about energy.

It's about understanding nutritional deficiencies. Simple carbohydrates, such as refined sugar, as opposed to complex carbohydrates (starch, fiber), pull essential nutrients out of the body. If you analyze unrefined sugar cane, besides sugar it also contains an array of B vitamins, minerals and enzymes, all of which are lost during processing. What's left is simple sugar, which is vitamin and mineral deficient. Now the body becomes deficient because it must supply the vitamins and minerals needed to digest, absorb and turn that sugar into energy.

The American Medical Association's Council on Food and Nutrition defines nutrition as "the science of food"—what is ingested, digested, absorbed, transported, utilized (turned into energy) and eliminated, via the lungs, urine and the bowel, and if these fail, the skin.

That's the whole point of this book. If food's not digested, it can't be absorbed and used.

And depriving your body of its primary energy source—carbohydrates—is not in the best interest of maintaining symptom-free, good overall health. Nor, as noted earlier, is the answer to be found in vitamin and mineral supplements.

Rather, the key to maintaining good overall health, and the prevention of chronic, degenerative diseases such as obesity, diabetes and heart disease, is in the essential compounds that are derived from the macronutrients—carbohydrates, proteins and lipids—that we consume every time we sit down at the dinner table.

Evolution of Nutritional Science

Our understanding of food and nutrition originated from the recognition in ancient times that certain foods changed how we felt. Some foods made us feel better and some made us feel worse; some foods made us warmer while others helped cool us down.

Eventually, the importance of carbohydrate, protein and fats became clear, as did the relationship of these macronutrients to energy production and growth and repair.

The next step in nutritional understanding came with the realization that there were micronutrients in food, and that the deficiency of one or more of those in a diet could lead to diseases, such as scurvy (vitamin C), anemia (iron), rickets (calcium and vitamin D), and pellagra (vitamin B), for example.

Fortunately, we seldom, if ever, see these conditions anymore, except in populations suffering extreme poverty.

Today, nutritional science is expanding into areas beyond vitamins and minerals, into bio-nutrients, such as isoflavones, which are plant-derived compounds with estrogenic activity. You can buy supplements touting the benefits of nitric oxide, which is an important cellular signaling molecule with a very short half-life of a few seconds in the blood.

Such advances are no doubt important, as we await explanations of how they can be used to maintain health.

Meanwhile, one scientific truth has become abundantly clear—that our inconvenient symptoms, which have not yet reached a chronic disease state, are caused by organs or tissues that are not able to adequately perform their intended functions necessary to maintain health. This may be caused by ongoing stress, be it structural stress, visceral stress or emotional stress.

If we can identify and reduce the stress, improve nutrition to those struggling organs, and improve waste removal, the body will resume normal function and the symptom or symptoms will be removed, or at least minimized.

Once, again, it's all about energy.

Once again, the body prefers carbohydrates as its primary source of energy, followed by protein and finally fats.

Interestingly, carbohydrates and protein-containing foods provide the same type of water-soluble vitamins—B and C. These are even called "stress vitamins." But each provides different minerals. Carbohydrates provide minerals that are alkaline in nature—sodium, potassium and magnesium. Protein provides acid elements, such as sulfur and phosphorus. This is a critical point when it comes to understanding your symptoms, and the deficiencies fueling them.

Are your symptoms being caused by a micronutrient or a macronutrient deficiency?

The next three chapters, starting with this one on carbohydrates, will deal consecutively with deficiency-related symptoms. Chapter 4 focuses on symptoms of protein deficiency; Chapter 5 on lipids.

So how would you know that your diet was responsible for your symptoms?

The following symptoms can all be related to problems in dietary choices, problems with digestion, absorption, transportation of nutrients, cellular utilization and energy production, or removal of waste products:

- Stiff, sore joints
- Headaches
- Heartburn
- Indigestion
- Gas pain and bloating
- Infrequent bowel movements (constipation)
- Frequent, soft bowel movements (diarrhea)
- Restlessness

- Irritability
- Feelings of anxiety
- Irregular sleep patterns

These are all non-specific symptoms—that is, you don't know whether they are related to carbohydrate, protein or fat deficiency. Or whether they are related to water-soluble or fat-soluble vitamin deficiencies. Or an alkaline mineral or acid element deficiency.

The answers to these questions will be found in this and the next two chapters.

What is a Carbohydrate?

The word *carbohydrate* is a very old term. It refers to a substance that contains carbon, as found in starch, sugars and fiber. Collectively, these are the body's preferred source of energy, with each requiring a separate digestive process.

Fiber is not supposed to be digestible. So, we'll talk about that last.

But first, how much carbohydrate do we need? That's a tough question.

What we do know is that diets with as little as 60 grams of carbohydrate will prevent the symptoms of starvation, and most authorities feel it is prudent not to go below 100 grams per day.

The most recent Dietary Guidelines for Americans recommends that carbohydrates make up 45 to 65 percent of your total daily calories. That means if you average 2,000 calories a day, between 900 and 1,300 calories should be from carbohydrates.

The Bottom Line

Even if you're consuming 100 grams of carbohydrates daily, you're going to wind up protein deficient, which means you're also going to wind up calcium deficient and susceptible to all the symptoms that go with that deficiency—cramps, aching bones, edema, and so on.

This brings us to the very top of the preferred fuel chain.

What is Starch?

Starch is the most common carbohydrate in the human diet. Major sources include cereals (rice, wheat, maize) and the root vegetables (potatoes, cassava).

There are two forms of starch in our diet—amylose and amylopectin. Depending on the plant, starch generally contains 20 to 25 percent amylose and 75 to 80 percent amylopectin. Amylose, when ingested, releases the simple sugars. Amylopectin, which occurs naturally in the cell walls of fruits and vegetables, increases the viscosity and volume of the stool and is helpful in preventing both constipation and diarrhea.

Before the advent of processed foods, people consumed large amounts of uncooked and unprocessed starch-containing plants, which are not easily digested. Microbes living within the large intestine can help break down these fibrous plants, releasing short-chain fatty acids that our bodies use, and which also support the maintenance and growth of the microbes themselves. (Some microbes are beneficial to us and others are not.)

We have a symbiotic relationship with these microbes living in our digestive system.

The highly processed foods in modern diets are more easily digested and release more glucose in the small intestine, which can then be absorbed and used by the body for energy.

Unfortunately, it is thought that this shift in energy delivery from raw, uncooked fruits and vegetables—complex carbohydrates—to processed foods may be contributing to the widespread development of metabolic disorders of modern life, including obesity and diabetes.

The enzymes that break down ("hydrolyze") starch into simple sugars for energy production are known as amylases. These starch-digesting enzymes are found in the plants themselves, in proportion to the amount of starch in each plant. Saliva is rich in amylase, and the pancreas also secretes this enzyme.

Such is Nature's design for the human body's preferred source of energy.

This preference was first brought to attention by the legendary Harvard physiologist Walter Bradford Cannon.

The Father of Physiology

Walter B. Cannon captured the medical world's imagination with his landmark theories, including the "flight or fight" response—a term he coined in 1915—and his expansion of Claude Bernard's concept of homeostasis, with respect to the body's ability to maintain constancy of glucose concentrations, body temperature, acid-base balance, and so on. All of this was set forth in Cannon's 1932 book, *The Wisdom of the Body,* published by W.W. Norton & Co., Inc., in New York.

Cannon pioneered the mixing of salts of heavy metals into foods in order to track them via X-ray technology through the digestive system. In doing so, he observed that food lies undisturbed in the upper part of the stomach after it enters from the esophagus. Dr. Edward Howell would later come to refer to this upper chamber as the "enzyme stomach," where salivary amylase goes to work predigesting starches.

But it was Cannon who observed early on that the peristaltic waves that move and mix the food start near the middle of the stomach and then deepen as they pass into the lower portion of the stomach. It is during this time that stomach acid initiates protein digestion by converting pepsinogen into the protein-digesting enzyme pepsin.

What Cannon ultimately concluded was that protein foods are discharged from the stomach more slowly than starch foods, but faster than fat.

He became the first to observe the body's preferences regarding energy production—carbohydrate first, then protein, then fats, which are the last to be digested.

Cannon also correctly concluded that protein empties more slowly than carbohydrate because it's being digested in the stomach, and that's what slows it down.

For those using stomach-acid blockers, if food in the stomach is not acidified, digestion of starch by salivary amylase continues in the stomach, while protein digestion is not initiated. We will discuss the ramifications of this in the next chapter, when we focus on proteins.

All in all, the balanced diet consists of real carbohydrate and good protein. Because the carbohydrate has the alkaline minerals and the protein has the acid minerals. Get them balanced and get them digested, and the body will take care of itself.

The key to understanding why the body lunges at starch is because it is so easy to digest for conversion into energy.

Which brings us to the quick fix.

Understanding Sugars

So what is a sugar?

When one thinks sugar (saccharide), one thinks sweet.

There are many chemical sugars, including some sweeteners we use that provide zero calories because the body does not make an enzyme to convert them to glucose, and they are therefore not absorbed. Diet food substitutes for sugar, such as aspartame and sucralose, are artificial non-saccharides.

Amylase digests (hydrolyzes, or breaks apart with water) starch, thus creating three types of simple sugars that the body can quickly convert to glucose for energy—if it can break them apart and absorb them.

Remember, salivary amylase works in the stomach and can even move starch and sugars into the small intestine before stomach acid is produced.

But it all starts with starch, which is a polysaccharide, or a long string of sugar molecules joined together. Add to this the digestive enzyme amylase and the starch is broken down into one of three separate disaccharides—lactose, which is derived from dairy, maltose from grains, and sucrose from most plants.

> The key to understanding sugar is: the body literally lunges at starch because it is so easy to digest, and because it creates sugar, for energy.

Water follows sugar. Where is the sugar? Is it staying in your bowel, or is it getting absorbed into your body? That's where the water is.

In the end, water follows the digested carbohydrates. If you've got water problems, regardless of where it is, sugar is involved. It's just a matter of figuring out which sugar is involved.

Digestion of Disaccharides to Monosaccharides

After salivary and pancreatic amylase has broken down the long-chain starch molecules into the three different disaccharides—lactose, maltose and sucrose—the next stage of digestion takes place. This occurs in the second part of the small intestine, the jejunum, where the molecules pass over hair-like projections called microvilli in which the sugar-digesting enzymes (disaccharidases) reside. These enzymes—lactase, maltase and sucrase—are produced on demand. In other words, the more sugar you consume, the greater the quantity of digestive enzymes the body is required to produce.

But there is a limit.

The body is only capable of producing what your genetic strength allows, and this includes enzyme production. Hence, it follows that no one can consume all the milk, grains or candy they desire.

And when the enzyme "well" runs dry, resulting in incomplete digestion, there are consequences—symptoms!

We become "intolerant," with an array of symptoms resulting from a failure to fully digest what we consume.

Excessive consumption of any of the three simple sugars will produce one of two possible symptom patterns. All three of these "intolerances" are commonly seen, but only two are recognized and identified by name. The third is a major national health problem that is hiding in plain sight.

Excessive lactose cannot be absorbed into the body and remains in the bowel causing painful gas and bloating. It pulls water from the body, causing very frequent, soft bowel movements (diarrhea).

Excessive maltose cannot be absorbed and, as a result, it also remains in the bowel, causing painful gas and bloating. And it too pulls water from the body causing frequent, soft bowel movements—i.e., diarrhea.

Sucrose, however, can be absorbed from the bowel into the body. Therefore, **excessive sucrose** moves across the gut wall and pulls water with it from the bowel. This causes gas and bloating and *infrequent* bowel movements, or constipation.

Again, if you've got water problems, sugar is involved. It's just a matter of figuring out which sugar is involved, because the water follows the sugar. Is it in the bowel? Is it in the body?

The symptoms associated with lactose or gluten intolerance are widely known. But not sucrose intolerance. Nobody in medicine tests for sucrose intolerance. Nobody tests urine to see if sucrose is leaving the body. Such testing is only done on newborns in the hospital to see if they have a genetic defect.

Yet, in society today, there is a much higher incidence of sucrose intolerance than either gluten or lactose intolerance.

And it isn't even on the radar of most primary care physicians or the public.

What are the symptoms of sucrose intolerance? Would you believe muscle weakness and an inability to concentrate, for starters?

Let's take a closer look at these three energy sources and the symptoms associated with excessive intake and/or the inability to digest what we do consume of each.

Sucrose

The "table sugar" or "granulated sugar" customarily used as a food is sucrose. It occurs naturally alongside fructose and glucose in fruits and some root vegetables, such as carrots. Differing proportions of sugars in these foods determines the range of sweetness we experience when we eat them.

White sugar is the pure, crystallized sucrose that has been extracted from either sugar cane or sugar beets. After harvesting, the juice is extracted from the vegetable source and boiled down to remove the molasses. As the moisture diminishes, the natural sucrose in the juice begins to crystalize. The crystallized sugar is then removed, leaving other extracts behind.

The key word here is "pure." Nutritionally speaking, what's left behind is the molasses, which is composed of 75 percent carbohydrate and 22 percent water. Molasses is also a rich source of vitamin B6 and several important minerals, including manganese, magnesium, iron, potassium and calcium, none of which are present in "pure" granulated sugar.

> I am reminded of a story I used to tell at my seminars. It was about a medical doctor from the state of Washington by the name of Rosalind Wulzen. Dr. Wulzen found that the nutrients in cane sugar—stress vitamins B and C, and alkaline minerals—were effective in relieving the symptoms in arthritis patients.

Dr. Wulzen contacted the sugar growers in Hawaii—this was just before Pearl Harbor—and she got them to can and send her the vitamin- and mineral-rich ingredients that they had removed in order to get the white sugar. What they canned and sent to her, however, never made it to the state of Washington because the cans exploded in the ship's hold midway across the Pacific. The cans, it turned out, also contained the plant enzymes from the sugar cane, which were doing their digestive work all the way over. Thus, the exploding cans!

Then the Japanese bombed Pearl Harbor, and Dr. Wulzen was forgotten.

It was at that point in my story that I took a fictional turn, describing to my seminar attendees how I had gone to Hawaii and contracted a man to take a job at the Dole Pineapple plant, sweeping the floors of all the stuff they had removed from the sugar, then putting it in a box—not a can—and sending it to me. I then brought in the National Enzyme Company—or so I told my audience—and we put that stuff in capsules, along with an appropriate enzyme formulation, for people with sore joints.

It was a prank. I never did contract anyone in Hawaii or call the National Enzyme Company about creating that product. But I made my point.

If you consume a lot of white sugar, and other refined sugar products, your body is going to become deficient in the stress vitamins and alkaline minerals it has to give up in order to deal metabolically with all that vitamin- and mineral-deficient sugar, and you are going to experience myriad symptoms associated with these deficiencies, including the constipation, stiff sore joints, heart arrhythmias and difficulty processing thoughts, which is associated with potassium deficiency, as well as the emotional issues associated with magnesium deficiency.

As a nation we are consuming an alarming amount of white sugar and other refined sugar additives. Back during the early 1800s, the average intake of sugar was only four to six pounds per person per year.

Things have changed.

Today it is estimated that the average person consumes approximately 100 pounds of refined sugar per year.

The U.S. Department of Agriculture puts sugar consumption at about 66 pounds per year by each American. However, when the USDA looked at refined sugar and corn sweeteners (i.e., high fructose corn syrup), the consumption estimate rose to 103 pounds per American per year.

There's a pattern here. In 1984, 45 percent of the calories in the American diet came from carbohydrate, while back in 1900 that percentage was 56 percent. However, during that same period the amount of refined sugar intake increased by more than 50 percent, while complex carbohydrate intake decreased by the same amount.

This is not a good pattern.

The concern is that we've become a nation of *sugarholics,* with children particularly at risk. The *U.S. Dietary Guidelines for Americans* recommends that people limit their total intake of added sugars and fats to 5 to 15 percent per day. Yet, University of California researchers point out, American children and adolescents get 16 percent of their total caloric intake from added sugars alone.

Sugar is a drug, not a food. And it has become a national addiction, whether it's coming from the 11 teaspoons in one 12-ounce can of soda, or fruit juice, or the 7 teaspoons in a single serving of yogurt.

Sugar is everywhere. It's an enormous industry with all kinds of government support and subsidies.

There's more.

Big Sugar?

The Chicago Tribune recently compared the sugar industry to Big Tobacco, noting that an industry rat study conducted more than four decades ago (that was never made public) found evidence linking sugar to heart disease and bladder cancer.

The sugar industry simply "pulled the plug on the study and buried the evidence." That's what senior researcher Stanton Glantz, director of the Center for Tobacco Control Research and Education at the University of California at San Francisco, told *The Tribune.*

Further rat studies with similar results were similarly shut down before they could be completed by withdrawal of industry funding, according to documents discovered by the University of California researchers. In these cases, rats fed a high sugar diet experienced increased blood levels of triglycerides, which contributes to cholesterol, and elevated levels of beta-gluturonidase, an enzyme associated with bladder cancer in humans.

There's more.

The same B vitamin and alkaline mineral deficiencies that occur with overconsumption of refined sugar, and the symptom patterns associated with these deficiencies, also appear when we consume too much white flour.

Bread was once the "staff of life." I was raised in a home where my father had decreed that bread would always be the first thing on the table and the last thing off. Every Saturday my maternal grandfather baked all the bread and rolls for the week for a large family. When my mother took me there, we could smell the aroma of baking bread a block away. I can still smell and taste the hot rolls smeared with fresh butter to this day.

Unfortunately, bread is not what it used to be, due to the lowering of mineral content by plant breeders and, to a much greater degree, to the refining of whole wheat to facilitate the extraction of white flour. Such milling, it has been noted by various sources, reduces vitamin B1 by 73 percent, vitamin B2 by 81 percent, vitamin B6 by 87 percent, vitamin E by 93 percent, calcium by 60 percent, magnesium by 85 percent, manganese by 86 percent, potassium by 77 percent, iron by 76 percent and zinc by 78 percent.

If only the refinement process were effective in restoring the original nutritional value. But you can't make graham crackers out of white bread.

What we see is the same array of symptoms with the consumption of white bread that we see with excess sugar consumption, because both are devoid (or near devoid) of B vitamins and alkaline minerals, and the body gives up these

B vitamins and alkaline minerals to digest them, resulting in the same deficiencies and the same mind-boggling array of symptoms that we see with excess sugar consumption.

Further, when white bread is digested, the end product is sugar.

So, the wheel comes full circle.

Which begs this question, we all know the symptoms of lactose and gluten intolerance. Why is it that nobody is aware of the more pervasive symptoms of sucrose intolerance?

All you have to do is look for the gas and bloating, and then see if the water is in the bowel or the body—in other words, are you experiencing diarrhea or constipation? The rest will sort itself out—the irritability; the stiff, sore joints; the inability to focus or to pay attention, and more.

It all comes down to how much sugar you are consuming compared to how much you can digest.

Now let's take a look at lactose.

Lactose

Lactose symptoms indicate one of two things, enzyme deficiency or excessive lactose ingestion above enzyme availability.

All human beings are lactose intolerant on a scale of zero to 100, based on the amount of lactose a person can take in and digest. Nobody is totally lactose intolerant, and nobody can drink all the milk they want to. All of us are somewhere in the middle, the closer you are to zero, the more often you will have symptoms.

It all comes down to this question: How much lactose are you taking in compared to how much lactase enzyme your body can produce to digest it?

And when you take in more than your enzyme capacity, the undigested lactose in your colon results in bacterial fermentation, producing hydrogen, carbon dioxide, and methane (sulfur) gases that cause the related excessive flatus, bloating and distention, and abdominal pain.

Lactase enzyme levels are high in newborns, permitting them to digest milk. These levels, however, decrease in the post-weaning period, rendering older children and adults unable to digest significant amounts of lactose.

That said, there is a genetic component to lactose deficiency, which affects 80 percent of blacks and Hispanics, and 90 percent of Asians, while 80 to 85 percent of whites of Northwest European descent produce lactase throughout life and are therefore able to digest milk and milk products.

Lactase deficiency resulting in lactose intolerance is also found in several conditions where damage has occurred to the mucosal lining of the small bowel. Among these conditions are: celiac disease, whereby the small intestine is hypersensitive to gluten; tropical sprue, a malabsorption disease commonly found in tropical regions, characterized by an abnormal flattening of the villi and inflammation of the intestinal lining; or acute intestinal infestations—i.e., bacterial overgrowth.

All these may be confused with irritable bowel syndrome (IBS) caused by other problems.

All told, most people recognize early in life that dairy products are a problem for them, and so they avoid eating dairy products. Symptoms typically require ingestion of more than the equivalent of 8 to 12 ounces of milk.

A child who cannot tolerate lactose develops diarrhea after ingesting significant amounts of milk and may not gain weight. An affected adult may have watery diarrhea, bloating, excessive flatus, nausea and abdominal cramps. Important here is that the diarrhea may be severe enough to purge other nutrients before they can be absorbed.

Other symptoms, such as rash, wheezing, or severe anaphylactic symptoms (particularly in children) suggest a cow's milk allergy.

Milk allergy is rare in adults.

Worth noting here is that a person can be slightly lactose intolerant. Or it's possible that your symptoms may be coming from some lactose mixed in with some gluten you're eating. If you're eating a bowl of Wheaties with milk on it and you think you are gluten intolerant, it may just be the lactose, or it may be a combination of both.

A gluten antibody test could help sort things out.

One thing is for certain. If you had the enzymes to handle the lactose, you'd be fine. The same is true for gluten.

Gluten Intolerance

Everybody knows what gluten intolerance is.

The symptoms, like those of lactose intolerance, include gas, bloating and diarrhea. And, like lactose intolerance, the reason for the diarrhea has to do with the need to move the undigested food out of the body. In other words, water is pulled out of the body and into the intestine to produce the diarrhea to flush it all away.

Gluten itself is a mixture of protein (gliadins) joined with starch and found in wheat and related grains, including barley, rye, oat and triticale. Gluten is the substance that gives elasticity to dough, helping it to rise and keep its shape. It also increases the bread's structural stability and contributes to its desirable chewiness.

Worldwide, gluten is used as a source of protein, both in foods prepared directly from sources containing it, and as an additive to foods otherwise low in protein.

Currently, there is a growing incidence of gluten-related disorders all around the world due to the progressive Westernization of diet, and an increased expansion of the Mediterranean diet, which includes a lot of foods that incorporate gluten. In recent years, new types of wheat with a higher amount of gluten peptides have been developed, some of which were found to be toxic, and this has prompted many countries to introduce gluten-free food products.

The gluten picture has become a complicated one, to say the least.

More than 250 symptoms of gluten "sensitivity" have been reported, including bloating, abdominal discomfort or pain, constipation and diarrhea, "brain fog," tingling and/or numbness in the hands and feet, fatigue, as well as muscular disturbances and bone or joint pain.

This wide range of overlapping symptoms makes the diagnosis of gluten sensitivity something of a task, and it's led to a lot of confusion. A recently developed blood test has been useful in some cases. It tests for an anti-gliadin antibody the body makes when a person fails to digest gluten—that is, the body is unable to separate the gliadin protein from the wheat product it is bonded to, resulting in an inability to digest maltose in the small intestine.

The diagnosis of gluten intolerance, the symptoms of which usually resolve with the elimination of gluten from the diet, involves distinguishing it from other gluten-related disorders, such as wheat allergy and celiac disease.

The whole issue of gluten intolerance, or non-celiac gluten sensitivity, like that of sucrose and lactose intolerance, may come down to the body's ability to produce the necessary enzymes to perform the digestive task at hand. In this case, the task is separating the gliadin proteins from the maltose they are bound to, so the starch can be digested and absorbed into the body.

This brings us to the one carbohydrate that cannot be digested—insoluble fiber.

Fiber

We cannot talk about fiber without fiber supplements coming to mind. The latest push is gummy supplements that you can chew. All these supplements do is add bulk to your stool, and that's how they're being marketed.

Of course, there's a lot more to fiber than simply keeping things moving.

The average adult eats only 15 grams of fiber per day, while the Institute of Medicine states that women need 25 grams of fiber per day and men need 38 grams. This recommended dietary intake of fiber is not via supplements. Eating more plant foods—i.e., vegetables, beans, fruit, whole grains—is the best way to consume fiber, according to the U.S. government's *2015 Dietary Guidelines.*

Experts insist that the human body cannot digest fiber because it does not produce cellulase, the enzyme needed to break down cellulose, and the main constituent of plant cell walls. If the cellulose is not broken down, the fiber cannot be digested. This is the reason why nutrition books promote cooking as a digestive aid—because it removes the cellulose. This is true. But you can also chew cellulose off the food you are eating.

In fact, there are two kinds of fiber—soluble and insoluble. Soluble fiber can be digested because it absorbs water. And the cellulase needed to digest the cellulose is contained in the vegetables we consume. All we have to do is chew these vegetables thoroughly to release the cellulase.

People who say, "I can't eat salads because they give me gas," are in fact failing to chew their vegetables thoroughly. If you do chew thoroughly, you will liberate the cellulase that is contained in the vegetables you are eating, and that cellulase will mix with your own salivary enzymes and predigest the cellulose in your stomach.

Soluble fiber is also digested by the friendly bacteria in your gut.

Insoluble fiber doesn't absorb water and neither you nor the plant have the enzymes to digest it.

This said, your body needs both soluble and insoluble fiber.

Foods rich in soluble fiber include oatmeal, nuts, beans, apples and blueberries. When you eat them raw, you can digest the soluble fiber down to its two components: glucose, for energy, and short-chain fatty acids. Since short-chain fatty acids are water-soluble, the body can put them to use as soon as they become available. They can be taken directly to the liver, or used as a source of nutrition for the cells in your colon.

Dietary fiber is not considered to be a source of calories, and yet the metabolites released by the bacteria in the colon are thought to be used by humans to meet their energy requirements. Short-chain fatty acids may provide roughly 10 percent of your daily calorie needs.

Consequently, they may also play an important role in maintaining health by reducing the risk of inflammation, Type II diabetes, obesity, heart disease and other conditions.

Short-chain fatty acids are also involved in the metabolism of not only lipids but carbohydrates as well.

So fiber is not just about adding bulk to your stools.

Insoluble fiber is found in the seeds and skins of fruit, as well as whole wheat bread and brown rice. Like soluble fiber, insoluble fiber can play a key role in controlling weight by staving off hunger pangs.

Eating lots of insoluble fiber also helps keep you regular, and if you become constipated, adding more insoluble fiber to your diet can get things moving. Since insoluble fiber is not digestible, it promotes the movement of material through your digestive system and increases bulk. Thus, it can be of benefit to those who struggle with constipation or irregular stools.

So how would you know if you're fiber deficient?

The most notable sign a person has a very low fiber intake is an increase in constipation. However, several negative physiological responses occur in individuals who consume low levels of dietary fiber over time, particularly an increased risk for coronary heart disease.

While there is a bountiful supply of fiber supplements available for purchase, which are all promoted to reduce gas, bloating and constipation, most experts recommend that fiber should be obtained through the consumption of fiber-containing foods because they contain the micronutrients (vitamins and minerals), not to mention the cellulase enzyme to digest them!

Which brings us back to vitamin and mineral supplements.

When it comes to determining what your deficiency is regarding the symptoms you are experiencing, it's not about vitamins and minerals. It's about the macronutrients (carbohydrates, proteins and lipids) and the essential compounds derived from them—i.e., hemoglobin, thyroxine, insulin, adrenaline and various hormones. Supplemental vitamins and minerals are not going to make essential compounds for you!.

Further, the days of vitamin deficiencies are long gone. As noted earlier in this book, vitamin deficiencies are identified as disease processes, such as scurvy and rickets. These disease processes were overcome with adequate food supply and public education many years ago.

Vitamins are still needed by the body, but in very small amounts. They are not needed in the huge amounts found in commercial vitamin supplements.

Moreover, most commercial vitamin and mineral supplements marketed as "natural" are not the same as vitamins and minerals appearing in various food sources. Rather, they are "synthetic" crystalized versions created by the pharmaceutical industry. They are made or processed with petroleum derivatives or hydrogenated sugars, intended to mimic the natural non-crystallized vitamins and minerals found in the foods we eat.

They are often advertised as "natural," but in most cases, there is nothing natural about them. Food-sourced vitamins and minerals have been shown to be far superior to their commercially produced counterparts.

Recent studies suggest that multivitamin and mineral supplements, which are used by 40 to 50 percent of men and women 50 years of age and older to the tune of $12 billion a year, have little or no impact on preventing chronic diseases, including cancer and heart disease, or reducing the risk for mental decline, such as memory loss or a "slowing down" in an individual's thinking abilities.

Some studies have even shown a slightly increased risk of heart disease and certain cancers despite "misleading commercials."

So what's the take-home message here?

First and foremost, it is important to recognize that vitamin and mineral supplements are not the key to relieving symptoms and maintaining health. Recent studies indicate, the best source of vitamins and nutrients we need are in the foods Nature put there in the first place—i.e., eating a balanced diet—and then making sure that we are digesting these foods and assimilating the essential compounds contained in them.

The Bottom Line

Vitamins and minerals do not perform work. The body's enzymes perform the necessary work to provide the body systems with the energy needed from the nutrients consumed.

---

is the key to preventing/relieving symptoms and ...₋.,.ning health.

With this in mind, let's move on to the body's principal sources of the critically important essential compounds that our bodies need, and the symptoms that result from their deficiency, starting with protein in Chapter 4.

Symptoms Related to Carbohydrate Metabolism

Carbohydrate Deficiency

Carbohydrates are the body's preferred source of food for energy production. Therefore, it follows that fatigue is the earliest sign. But, when the body has to resort to converting amino acids for energy it also loses water and dryness of various tissues soon becomes evident.

- Dry mouth, nose, or eyes
- Muscle weakness
- Easily startled
- Inability to concentrate
- Difficulty swallowing and voice affected by stress

Poor Carbohydrate Digestion

There are several steps in digestion of carbs, starting with chewing of fibrous foods. Starch digestion is easily accomplished, but the digestion of simple sugars is problematic and not easily diagnosed.

- History of lactose or gluten intolerance
- Craving or thirst for cold liquids or foods
- Intolerance of dairy products, grains, or sugar
- Sensitive to air pollutants, such as perfumes, smoke, etc
- Tolerates stress very poorly

Inadequate Stomach Acid

Carbohydrate digestion is not dependent on stomach acid, but inadequate protein digestion leads to increased use of foods high in white sugar and flour.

- History of pernicious anemia
- Loss of taste for meat
- Strong desire to eat when not hungry
- Indigestion, particularly 2 to 3 hours after eating
- Flatulence – lower bowel gas

Gas, Bloating and Bowel Distension

This troublesome symptom can have many causes and often begins with inadequate chewing of foods and increased use of foods high in refined sugars and flour.

- History of chronic gas, bloating, and distention
- Unusual fullness after eating
- Craving or thirst for cold liquids or foods
- Avoidance of raw food, especially vegetables
- Rapid ingestion of food without chewing food completely

Early Symptoms Related to the Kidneys

- History of reactive hypoglycemia
- Suffer from airborne allergies
- Dark circles under the eyes
- Nausea/vomiting (e.g., morning sickness of pregnancy)
- Muscular low back pain

Alkaline Mineral (Potassium) Deficiency

Ingestion of excess simple sugars, primarily sucrose, requires increased amounts of dietary alkaline minerals and vitamin C and B complex. Symptoms result when they become inadequate. Would you describe yourself as:

- Type A personality, for example, driven and aggressive
- endency to problems of indigestion and constipation
- Stiff joints, especially after rest, loss of mobility
- Sensitive to sudden sounds, startles easily
- Headaches in back of head and neck

Alkaline Mineral (Magnesium) Deficiency

Magnesium is more directly related to structural and emotional symptoms than potassium. Both gradually become deficient on a diet high in refined carbohydrates.

- History of injury to tailbone
- Restlessness or insomnia
- Inability to concentrate; has daydreams or has nightmares.
- Unresolved health problems
- Painful tailbone, hurts to sit down

Deficiency of Water-Soluble "Stress" Vitamins

- History of low blood pressure problems
- Wake up after sleeping a few hours and cannot go back to sleep
- Dizziness or lightheadedness, especially when bending over
- Suffer from frequent nightmares or panic attacks
- Frequent mood swings, feeling "blue" or melancholy

Chapter 4

Protein

Carbohydrates provide the body with the energy it needs, and protein does that plus a whole lot more. While carbohydrates are used exclusively for energy production, **protein is your life's blood, and its deficiency is at the bottom of most chronic degenerative diseases.**

Proteins, from the Greek word *protos,* meaning *primary* or *first,* are large, naturally occurring biomolecules consisting of one or more chains of amino acids, which are made up of carbon, hydrogen, oxygen and nitrogen atoms, as well as sulfur and other elements, such as iron and phosphorous.

Without question, protein is the major player in the field of macronutrients. Carbohydrates and lipids are important for sure, with each having important roles, and all three can be converted into energy when needed.

But it is protein—and only protein—that plays the dual role of providing nutrients and maintaining normal function within the extracellular fluids that make up the internal environment of your body, and this includes blood. It is these extracellular fluids that deliver nutrients to cells and remove their metabolic waste products for elimination through the kidneys and lungs, and the skin when necessary.

Protein pretty much runs this show, from the production of micronutrients that nourish and fuel the body cells, to the transport of these nutrients throughout the body, to the elimination of metabolic waste products, and finally the maintenance of this extracellular environment—regulating water volume, maintaining pH levels and more.

Carbohydrates are the body's first source of fuel when it comes to meeting energy needs because starch is swiftly broken down in the stomach by salivary enzymes. Carbs are the quick fix. The problem is, only a small amount is stored in the liver for rapid conversion to glucose. It is true that the muscles store glucose in a form that can be quickly used for "fight or flight," but they cannot share that glucose with the rest of the body.

Protein is the backup energy source when the body is under stress, be it emotional, visceral or structural.

The brain, sensing it does not have adequate glucose to meet its energy demands, starts pulling stored amino acids from the cells and sending them to the liver for conversion into glucose. If this continues beyond the short term, protein deficiency symptoms will kick in—swelling in the hands and feet, cold hands and feet, muscle cramps at night, menstrual cramps, hot flashes, bleeding gums and the inability to tolerate exercise.

That's just the short list.

The Bottom Line

Proteins are essential for all living things. Proteins must therefore be included in the diet in ample amounts to sustain life.

There are two ways of looking at protein's contribution to overall health. One is the functions of dietary proteins; the other is the functions of plasma proteins. Let's start by looking at the functions of dietary proteins.

Dietary Proteins

On the dietary side, protein has a role in growth and tissue repair, formation of essential body compounds, and antibody formation.

1. **Growth or Increase in Muscle Mass.** This is possible when there is an appropriate mixture of amino acids over and above the amount needed for maintenance (homeostasis) and the repair of tissue. Some cells require larger amounts of specific amino acids. For example, hair, skin and nails require larger amounts of the sulfur-containing amino acids found in animal protein.

   Hence, women who struggle with hair, skin and nail problems are usually sulfur deficient, which goes back to protein. Sulfur is also needed for cartilage repair.

2. **Formation of Essential Body Compounds.** Whenever there is a protein deficiency, these essential compounds receive priority over other less important protein functions. Hormones such as insulin, epinephrine (which you may know as adrenaline), and thyroxin are all proteins. Hemoglobin and almost all of the factors involved in blood clotting are also proteins. The photoreceptors in the eye that are responsible for vision are proteins, as are the brain's neurotransmitters dopamine (the alertness chemical) and serotonin (the calming chemical).

Once again, homeostasis comes first, followed by the formation of these essential body compounds. Without adequate protein, these essential compounds begin to suffer.

When the body is under stress, it's using a lot of epinephrine (adrenaline). How long can this go on if you're protein deficient?

It takes eight days for the body to incubate thyroxin. When a person is under major stress for an extended period of time, thyroxin supplies diminish to the point where the person needs medical intervention, and perhaps a pharmaceutical version of the thyroid hormone.

Then remember there's dopamine, the alertness chemical, and serotonin, the calming chemical.

All of these essential compounds suffer in times of protein deficiency.

3. **Finally, There's Antibody Formation.** Protein deficiency accounts for a large amount of infant mortality among malnourished children (in impoverished areas) because specific antibodies against infection cannot be formed.

Food for thought: if a woman is protein deficient when she becomes pregnant, she is probably going to be protein deficient throughout her pregnancy, as the demands of the baby must be met.

Taking in the bigger picture, think about how many chronic immune problems there are in the world today that modern research continues to explore.

Plasma Proteins

The proteins that reside in the blood, the plasma proteins, are responsible for maintaining homeostasis. They are not used by cells to facilitate energy production, growth or repair. Plasma proteins are made in the liver; their sole purpose is to maintain homeostasis.

For plasma proteins, these tasks include: the maintenance of acid/alkaline balance (pH), regulation of water balance, transport of nutrients and waste, and the removal of toxic compounds.

Looking at each of these functions, we learn about the following:

1. **Acid/Alkaline Balance.** The body's work to maintain an acid/alkaline balance is a behind-the-scenes struggle that goes on 24/7 without us even being aware of it. Plasma proteins are buffers that have the ability to neutralize both excess acid and alkali in the blood, thus maintaining a normal acid-base balance. The blood has to be maintained within a certain narrow limit of pH. Any deviation can mean a trip to the emergency room.

2. **Regulation of Water Balance.** Plasma proteins are like magnets. They attract water and hold it in solution. Water moves towards protein. It's that simple. Just as protein holds water inside the shock-absorbing intravertebral discs, plasma protein molecules prevent water from leaking out of the blood into the tissues, keeping the critical "osmotic" balance that is key to maintaining homeostasis. The accumulation of fluid in the tissues is

an early warning sign of protein deficiency. Excess fluid gives tissues a soft, spongy, bloated appearance, as in the case of a protein deficiency and bloating that comes with menstruation. The maintenance of water balance in the body is critical.

In 2007, a 28-year-old California woman died after taking part in a water drinking contest held by a radio station. This woman drank so much water that her extracellular fluids became diluted and excessively low in sodium and other electrolytes, compared to the fluids inside her body cells. As a result, extracellular water began forcing its way into the woman's cells, to balance the concentration. This caused her brain to swell up, and she died.

Extremes aside, it's protein that maintains the delicate day-to-day extracellular and intracellular water balance in our bodies.

3. **Transport of Nutrients and Waste.** Sodium plays an essential role in the transport of nutrients across the intestinal wall into the blood. Yet it is protein that moves nutrients from the blood to the tissues, and across the cell membranes into the cell. Most of the transportation of nutrients to the cells and waste from the cells to the kidneys and lungs is done by plasma proteins:

   • Calcium is carried by protein
   • Iron is carried by protein
   • Cholesterol is carried by protein
   • Hormones are carried by protein

And so it follows, when there is an inadequate supply of protein, less of these carrier proteins are available, and the transportation of nutrients and the removal of cellular waste products can eventually become impaired, and with it, homeostasis.

4. **The Role of Proteins in the Removal of Toxic Compounds.** For plasma proteins, this task involves attaching to the toxic substances and transporting them to the kidney. It's then up to the kidney to sort out what to keep in the body and what to eliminate. As for the detoxification process itself, this is performed primarily by enzymes (a.k.a. proteins) found in the liver.

Again, one would be hard pressed to find anything taking place in the body that does not involve the conspicuously oversized, all-important protein molecule.

So how much protein does your body need every day to stay healthy? This is where the importance of dietary protein is often understated. While some athletes and bodybuilders consume large amounts of protein in an attempt to "muscle up," the rest of us are often told that we are eating too much protein, which is too often not the case.

Recommended Dietary Allowances for Macronutrients

The Recommended Dietary Allowance (RDA) is the amount of a nutrient you need to meet your basic nutritional requirements. It represents the minimum amount you need to keep from getting sick. It does not mean this is the specific amount you are supposed to eat every day.

The generally accepted daily allowance for protein is 0.8 grams per kilogram of bodyweight, with men requiring slightly more protein than women. This can be found in any nutritional textbook.

To determine your RDA for protein, multiply your weight in pounds by 0.36, or use the USDA's online calculator. Let's say you are a 30-year-old female leading a sedentary lifestyle, not pregnant, and not on birth control medication. Roughly, you would need about 50 grams of protein per day, which translates to 1.6 ounces. A male leading the same sedentary lifestyle would require 2.0 ounces to avoid a deficiency.

This translates roughly to as little as 10 percent of the total daily calories for a relatively active adult. In comparison, the average American consumes around 16 percent of their daily calories in the form of protein, from both plant and animal sources.

However, experts point out, these recommendations are based on the requirements of the average person leading a sedentary lifestyle, and they do not take into account the use of protein for energy under stress.

And there's more.

For those who continue to believe we eat too much protein, I call your attention to a June 2015 conference in Washington, D.C. The conference was attended by 40 nutrition scientists to discuss research on protein and human health. Their findings were published in a special supplement to the June 2015 issue of the *American Journal of Clinical Nutrition*. In it, the Protein Summit experts argue that 16 percent is anything but excessive. In fact, the reports suggest that Americans may eat too little protein, not too much. The potential benefits of higher protein intake, they argue, include preserving muscle strength despite aging, and maintaining a lean, fat-burning physique.

Some studies described in the summit reports suggest that protein is more effective if you space it out over the day's meals and snacks rather than loading up at dinner like Americans do.

> Based on the totality of the research presented at the summit, the experts estimate that taking up to twice the RDA of protein is a safe and good range to aim for. This equates roughly to 15 to 25 percent of total daily calories, although it could be above or below this range, depending on your age, sex, and your activity level.

This fits nicely into the recommendation from the current Dietary Guidelines for Americans, that we get 10 to 35 percent of daily calories from protein.

Finally, when it comes to dietary recommendations, there are no average people. There are so many variables that come into play. For instance, young individuals need more protein for growth. Bone formation is not complete until age 20, or thereabouts. Older people need to reduce their calories, but not protein.

What is your lifestyle? Do you lead a sedentary life, with light exercise, such as regular walking, or do you have a more extensive workout routine?

How much stress do you encounter during the day? This is a widely misunderstood concept. Again, we're not just talking about mental stress. It can be structural stress, relating to an individual's daily struggle to remain upright in a world governed by the force of gravity, or it can refer to visceral or emotional stresses, all of which can require more nutrition.

Do you drive a beer truck? Do you spend your days hauling heavy cases of beer in and out of stores all day long, or are you a stay-at-home mom raising children and maintaining a household, or an empty nester?

Maybe you are a tournament chess player, perhaps? You'd be surprised how much energy you can use during a chess tournament. I speak from experience. I learned how to play chess at a boy's club when I was 10 years old, though I didn't play in my first tournament until I was 38, when an attorney friend dragged me up to a weekend tournament 45 miles from where I was practicing. I didn't think either one of us had any business entering this tournament, but he was insistent.

The way these tournaments are set up, each player has 2 hours to make 40 moves. You play three games on Saturday. Then you come back for two more games on Sunday.

If you win your first game, you go up against a tougher opponent. If you lose, you go up against another person who has lost. That's how it goes through the five games.

In my first game I was up against a pretty good player. He was a college professor. I got a draw with him. I was amazed, and so was he. Next, I was up against a tougher player and won!

Next I'm up against an even tougher player. He was my brilliant Japanese friend. The sun was going down and we were sitting there in the middle of the game when all of a sudden it hit me. I couldn't process thought. My mind went blank. I knew who I was, I knew where I was, I was looking at the board, but I couldn't process thought. I sat there for several minutes with him looking at me and finally I tipped my King over, which means you're resigning.

"Howard," he said, "you don't have to do that. I'm winning, but not by much."

"You don't understand," I told him. "I can't think."

And he said, "You haven't played in a tournament for a long time. You're not really in shape, are you?"

That's what happens when you run out of mental energy and you're not able to process meaningful thought.

That's the only time that ever happened to me in my entire life. I had worked so hard that day—10 hours of constant mental processing. You have to be in shape for those things.

The Bottom Line

The brain is a glucose hog and my glucose was all used up. There was no place left in my body to go for it.

I went home that night and had visions of chessboards in my head. I had two more games left to play on Sunday. I had a good breakfast and managed to struggle through them.

But that was quite a learning experience. I was just bringing nutrition into my practice, and I quickly came to realize in a very profound and personal way that being a chess tournament player was by no means a typical "sedentary" lifestyle, and that there are many ways in which the body uses up energy, with carbohydrates first, followed by protein, and finally stored fat.

But by the time you go through protein and get around to burning fat, you're in trouble if it continues long term.

Hence the importance of consuming adequate daily protein. This amount varies from person to person. There's no such thing as typical.

The RDA for protein goes right out the window the moment a woman becomes pregnant, or when she starts nursing her newborn child.

Or when she is menstruating.

Menstruation means a woman is discharging blood and other material from the lining of the uterus. Menstrual blood contains blood cells and hemoglobin (iron and protein), in addition to the corpus luteum (lining of the uterus), which must be created every month if a woman doesn't get pregnant. The corpus luteum, like most body tissues, contains protein and reproductive hormones.

Why are there no specific dietary recommendations for menstruating women? We are told they must get enough iron in their diet, but what about protein?

Again, there's no such thing as typical.

Which Brings us to PMS or Premenstrual Syndrome

Women had been coming to me with PMS from the day I opened my practice back in the late 1960s. It was a big problem then, as it is now. In an effort to get a handle on the source of their symptoms, I began offering a free 24-hour urinalysis to any PMS patient who would agree to collect it. What I found was that these women didn't have enough calcium coming out in their urine on a daily basis during the month. You're supposed to lose a certain amount of calcium every day. This has been known and documented for well over 100 years. These women were not losing calcium, which told me they were calcium deficient and the body was holding onto what calcium it had.

It made sense, because calcium is necessary to prevent tetany—muscle spasms or muscle cramps. Furthermore, when a person becomes calcium deficient, they are subject to mood disturbances, such as irritability and anxiety, as well as insomnia or irregular sleep patterns—all PMS symptoms. Some of this can also be due to a related deficiency in serotonin, which is a calming neurotransmitter.

However, the calcium deficiency was not the real culprit. The urine tests also revealed these women were voiding excess alkalinity. This suggested to me that they were protein deficient, because protein is responsible for buffering excess alkalinity. Protein is also responsible for maintaining the amount of calcium a person has in their blood.

Calcium exists in the blood in two forms—free-floating calcium and calcium that is bonded to protein. The ratio of free-floating calcium to calcium bound to protein—approximately 50/50—must never change if homeostasis is to be maintained. As protein levels go down in the blood, so does calcium.

Because homeostasis within the extracellular fluid must be maintained at all costs, the blood-test levels of protein (albumin) will usually appear normal in these cases. However, due to the energy deficiency, amino acids inside the individual cells are being sent to the liver for conversion to glucose. At that point, symptoms of protein deficiency appear.

So while the women I was testing appeared to be calcium deficient, they were in fact protein deficient.

Furthermore, protein attracts water. When a person becomes protein deficient, in addition to calcium, water also leaves the blood. When water leaves the bloodstream, it collects in the tissues, which results in the edema, or bloating, women experience during their menstrual cycle.

So, it all comes down to protein deficiency. The fact that PMS is not a disease is why pharmacology has failed to help women with PMS symptoms, with hot flashes, and so on. The only way to restore normal function in such cases is by giving the body the nutrition it needs in order to function normally.

At least 95 percent of my female patients during the course of my clinical practice were protein deficient at the cellular level.

Then there's **osteoporosis,** demineralization of bone. While it is a medical condition there can be an underlying nutritional component. Bone is made up of protein, calcium and phosphorous. Demineralization can begin early with a protein deficiency and progress unrecognized for years, ending with the chronic degenerative process that is finally recognized as osteoporosis.

Then there's **anemia**. In my practice, most of the female patients I saw who said they were anemic were not actually iron-deficient. They were protein deficient.

The Bottom Line

The body needs adequate protein to function normally, and certain lifestyles may impede your ability to get that protein, and the essential amino acids your body requires.

Are you a vegetarian? It is important to know that plant proteins are incomplete proteins, in the sense that individual plants do not contain all the essential amino acids that our bodies require but do not have the ability to synthesize. The nine amino acids we humans cannot synthesize are: phenylalanine, valine, threonine, tryptophan, methionine, leucine, isoleucine, lysine and histidine.

These we must get from the foods we eat.

True vegetarians must be very careful to mix and match the vegetables they eat to get all the different types of amino acids they need to maintain health. It can be done, but you really have to know what you are doing to get a balanced amino acid picture, using combinations of foods, such as corn and beans, soybeans and rice, or red beans, which are a better source of amino acids.

The essential amino acids with the lowest level of availability in the American diet are valine and tryptophan. Foods rich in valine include dairy products, grains, meat, mushrooms, peanuts and soy protein. High tryptophan foods include turkey, nuts, seeds, cheese, red meat, chicken, fish, oats, beans, lentils and eggs.

Then there's tyrosine, which is nonessential because the body is able to manufacture it from phenylalanine, which is found in a variety of protein-rich foods, such as beef and soy, and green leafy vegetables, especially spinach. Symptoms of tyrosine deficiency include: flu-like symptoms, unexplained weight gain, poor temperature regulation, low blood pressure, vocal hoarseness, dry skin, constipation, and brittle hair or fingernails. Women with tyrosine deficiency may experience abnormally heavy menstrual periods due to low thyroid hormone levels. Good sources of tyrosine include milk, cheese, yogurt and cottage cheese, along with legumes (beans and peanuts).

Some vegetarians become "ovo-tarians," incorporating eggs, which are by far the best source of protein (complete balanced amino acid content) on the planet.

Many young women I encountered during the course of my practice considered themselves to be vegetarians when in reality they were what I called "pasta-tarians." They were eating pasta to avoid meat. For the record, neither pasta nor white rice or wild rice are good sources of essential amino acids.

Further, the way the body uses amino acids is not helter-skelter, but rather a very delicate orchestration, making supplementation a rather complicated affair, to say the least.

Think of the hypothalamus as the conductor of an amino acid orchestra consisting of 30 violins, 12 cellos, 10 double basses, an assortment of woodwind instruments, four flutes, four oboes, four clarinets, four bassoons, and a full percussion section, with one lone musician alternating between cymbals and the triangle, who God forbid should miss his cue.

Back in the 1970s, they were going to transform medicine by using individual amino acids. We'll give you phenylalanine if you have arthritis, they said. But it didn't work. Because the hypothalamus said, "I don't need any more violins. I don't care how good he is. I don't need him."

Again, 95 percent of my female patients over the years turned out to be protein deficient. Most of the health care practitioners I have examined who were on raw food diets or vegan diets, because they believe philosophically that this is the healthiest way to go, are protein deficient.

If you are going to pursue a vegetarian diet, you need to consume adequate and balanced sources of protein.

Finally, there are the vegetarians who ask themselves, why not become a fruitarian? The answer to that question is simple, because fruits do not contain nitrogen, and nitrogen-deficient is one of the last things you want to become.

> Protein is the body's sole source of nitrogen. Maintaining a positive nitrogen balance is the optimal state for muscle growth.

That means the **nitrogen** intake from protein is greater than the **nitrogen** output from protein utilization. This is the **body's** anabolic state and is necessary for growth, and life itself.

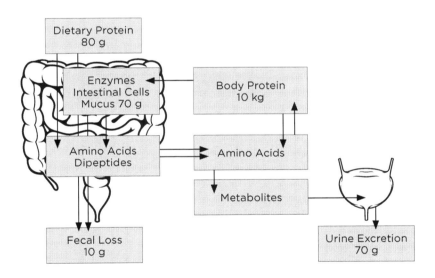

When we talk about a young, growing child in a positive nitrogen balance, we are saying that nitrogen is essential for that growth. As we age, we gradually move towards a negative nitrogen balance. This means we do not require as much nitrogen for growth, but we certainly need protein for repair

WHAT IS YOUR NUTRITIONAL DEFICIENCY?

of tissues and to maintain normal functions. Remember, only protein contains essential nitrogen, not carbohydrates and fats. Studies show that as we age we still require protein, but often our ability to digest and metabolize protein is gradually diminished. In other words, without protein a person cannot live for long.

Thus, one cannot become a fruitarian and stay healthy for very long.

Best Sources of Protein

So, what are the best sources for protein?

The very best source of dietary protein, bar none, is eggs. Seafood is an excellent source of protein, as well as white-meat poultry, milk, cheese, yogurt, and lean beef.

On the vegetarian side, there's quinoa, edamame, chia seeds, lentils, tempeh, chickpeas, peanut butter, beans and soy. Worth noting, one-half cup of beans contains as much protein as an ounce of broiled steak.

All this assumes, as noted earlier, that you are digesting what you are consuming—that your body's enzyme potential is up to par.

It also assumes that you are not using acid-blocking or antacid medications that would impede your body's ability to digest protein. Long-term use of these medications puts you at high risk of becoming protein deficient.

What's more, if you double your protein intake when you are not fully digesting it because you are on long-term acid-blocking medications, this could cause major problems.

That said, a person is not going to know they are protein deficient until they develop symptoms. Blood tests are not the answer, because the body's number one priority is to maintain homeostasis, and the blood tests hospitals use to measure the amount of protein in the blood will always come up normal, until you're really sick. There are several other ways to recognize a protein deficiency—for example, a 24-hour urine sampling.

A protein deficiency also can be diagnosed by a hands-on examination by a health care provider who is trained in uncovering nutritional deficiencies by tracking involuntary muscle contractions to their visceral source, or sources. This can be a complicated process, in some cases involving multiple nutritional deficiencies and multiple organ systems.

What to Watch For

What are the warning signs of protein deficiency? What symptoms suggest that you are not consuming or digesting adequate amounts of protein to meet your body's needs?

- **Craving Sweets.** Again, when you run low on carbohydrates for energy, your body turns to protein for conversion into glucose. That is why people under chronic stress are protein deficient. You might think the body would crave high-protein foods, but no, it wants the "quicker fix." It's not going for the hamburger, it's going for the bun. It wants sugar, and it wants it now!

- **Fatigue.** This is the most common complaint voiced by patients entering a doctor's office. Fatigue has many causes, one of which can be protein deficiency. It's all about energy. Your body is struggling to maintain homeostasis in the midst of ongoing structural, visceral and emotional challenges, and you don't have enough protein for energy. And let's not forget iron. You've got to have protein to transport iron, and to absorb it, or you're going to become anemic.

- **Swelling of the Hands and Feet.** Edema, or water gain, which appears as a collection of fluid under the skin, most commonly affects the legs, feet, and ankles. As we've seen in women with PMS, one of the important functions of protein is to maintain water in the blood. Protein is a magnet for water. When you are protein deficient, water will leave the blood and collect in the tissues. Another tell-tale sign of a protein deficiency is increased water secretions coming from your mouth, nose or eyes. Again, protein is the magnet, and when you are protein deficient, you can lose water. It's that simple.

- **Cold Hands and Feet.** This again is related to protein holding water in the blood. As water is lost, the warming effect that full blood circulation provides is reduced.

- **Muscle Tension Headache.** I have found that in many cases, these chronic, recurring headaches can involve a digestive problem caused by an energy deficiency when carbohydrates are used up and the body starts converting protein for energy. The organs 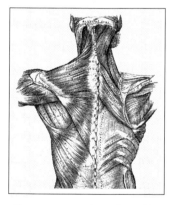 of digestion are innervated from the nerves leaving the spine in the middle of the thoracic spine, between the shoulder blades. Imagine an inverted pyramid. A muscle, the trapezius, runs from the spine in the area of the kidneys upward and over the shoulder blades to the outward points of the shoulders, and then up to the base of the skull. If there is any visceral dysfunction, involving the kidney, digestive, or other organs that share innervation with this muscle, the resulting involuntary muscle contraction pulling on the base of the skull will eventually produce a headache.

- **Skin Rashes.** Most skin rashes, which may or may not be accompanied by dry or flaking skin, can be a symptom of a protein deficiency. More involved rashes, such as dermatitis, eczema and psoriasis, have more complicated issues and will be discussed in the next chapter.

More complicated issues are inevitable with protein-related symptoms. This stems from the fact that protein has important homeostatic relationships with other nutrients, such as calcium, sulfur, magnesium, phosphorus, iron, cholesterol, vitamin C and the entire vitamin B complex.

Consider the following:

- **Anxiety, Irritability, Restlessness.** As discussed earlier in this chapter, anxiety and restlessness are associated with the protein-calcium bond, with a deficiency in protein leading to a deficiency in blood-borne calcium. This relationship also accounts for muscle cramps, menstrual cramps, and difficulty tolerating exercise, which may be related to stiff, sore joints.

- **Stiff, Sore Joints.** Protein, calcium and phosphorous have relationships with each other. There's a balance between protein and calcium, and a balance between calcium and phosphorous. All three make up bone. If you are deficient in any of these, protein being the key, you've got stiff, sore joints. Do you have frequent writer's cramp, or are you a slow starter in the morning? This is most often associated with the protein and phosphorus relationship.

ling or Brittle Hair.** Hair is made up of protein and ific amino acids that contain sulfur. Hence, a deficiency lead to your hair lacking the amount of sulfur it needs to stay healthy.

- **Ridges in Fingernails.** Sulfur is also needed in the fingernails. Furthermore, white lines or spots in the fingernails and toenails can be caused by a lack of protein and zinc in the diet. Zinc is involved in 40 different metabolic enzymes in the human body. **According to nutrition experts, the entire human race is borderline zinc deficient.**

- **Difficulty Sleeping.** This can be caused by a serotonin deficiency, which in turn can be caused by a lack of the amino acid tryptophan. The absence of serotonin is often responsible for the inability to relax, to become serene, and to drift off to sleep easily. The lack of specific minerals like potassium and magnesium may also result in the inability to sleep.

- **Slow Healing.** Patients who do not heal or rebound quickly after an illness or injury are often protein deficient. The body needs protein to repair tissue. Amino acids, the building blocks of protein, are crucial to this process.

- **Unexplained Weight Loss.** This always involves protein. In the case of muscle wasting, the body is actually breaking down muscle tissue to get at protein. Invariably, this indicates something very serious requiring immediate medical attention, such as a cancer that is using the body's protein to facilitate its own exponential growth.

That's the laundry list.

The signs and symptoms of protein deficiency are indeed many and varied, with a lot of overlap when it comes to related deficiencies of essential vitamins and minerals. This made for some very tricky trial-and-error diagnoses on my own part, as I pursued this winding learning curve.

So, is this you?

Is any of this you? It's certainly worth pondering.

Now let's move on to lipids.

Chapter 5

Lipids

This book is all about figuring out what your deficiency is. We have been very careful to point out that it is not about vitamins and minerals, but rather the macronutrients—carbohydrate, protein and lipids, in that order—that provide the fuel to run the body's organs. **Regardless of what your symptoms are, the deficiency is always energy.**

What is needed is a way to identify the organ system that is unable to function adequately and fulfill its role in maintaining homeostasis, and then provide that struggling organ system with the energy it needs to do its job before the body reaches a "disease state."

It's all about maintaining homeostasis within the extracellular fluids, including the blood, so that nutrients can be delivered to the body's cells, and waste can be picked up and eliminated. It's all about maintaining normal levels of everything from cholesterol, glucose and uric acid, to water volume. If you have too much water in your body fluids, you will have high blood pressure; too low, and you will have low blood pressure.

Too much or too little of anything, and your body will not be maintaining normal function. We've seen all this in action in earlier chapters.

It takes energy for each body organ to maintain homeostasis, and normal function.

It's all about energy!

We have proceeded through the macronutrients, beginning with carbohydrate, which is the body's preferred source for energy because sugar is so readily and easily absorbed. The body also has a unique way of moving starch right through the stomach, past protein and fat, and into the duodenum where the pancreatic enzymes can go to work on it ASAP. This is not in dispute. As noted earlier, Walter Cannon laid this all out back in 1896. It's accepted science.

When it comes to energy, carbohydrate is the preferred fuel.

The body's use of carbohydrate or protein for energy is perfectly normal. However, in this chapter we leave normal function. When the body is in a state of chronic stress, whether it's structural, visceral or emotional stress, it is then forced to resort to stored fat for energy. This is why the body stores fat—for emergency energy when it has used up its carbohydrate and protein sources.

The body's ability to turn to stored fat is wonderful in an emergency situation, or when it enables a mother to carry her newborn baby up and down the stairs and around the house and down the street. But it's not wonderful when the body must turn to stored lipids to deal with chronic, unremitting stress, be it structural, visceral or emotional in nature. It's at this point that the wheels begin to fall off the wagon. And it's all downhill from here unless this situation is remedied.

Let's take a look at the Big Picture.

What follows is a list of some general symptoms one may experience when the body is continually using fat for energy. Under chronic stress there is a natural progression through your organ systems, and I have organized the symptoms this way. However, please do not make decisions regarding your health without talking them over with your health care provider.

Let's Start with Diet

Is your diet providing your body with all the energy it needs?

When you're under chronic stress, your body winds up using lipids as an energy source. This results in lipid and steroidal hormone deficiencies, which in turn results in reproductive problems.

> If lipids are going to be used on a continued basis for energy production, the body will not be able to produce adequate reproductive (steroidal) hormones, which, besides resulting in infertility issues for both sexes, are responsible for an array of non-pathological symptoms that appear monthly and have plagued women since the beginning of time. For more information, refer to my book, *The Enzyme Advantage for Women,* published in 2016 in paperback.

For men, inadequate reproductive hormones can mean low sperm counts, or immature sperm counts, leading to possible birth defects.

A woman is not going to be able to function well without adequate reproductive hormones, whether she wants to have children or not. Being able to balance estrogen and progesterone is critical for a woman's health and well-being. If you are under chronic stress and using fat for energy, you ɔing to be able to balance hormones adequately; and ɔe subject to all the "female" symptoms associated nonal imbalance.

Further, when the body starts converting fat for energy, blood triglycerides go up and insulin production slowly goes down, putting one on a course to metabolic syndrome and Type II diabetes.

Lipids are also used to produce the myelin sheath insulation for the body's nerves, the deterioration of which can result in nerve irritation and, in the long run, a host of neurodegenerative autoimmune diseases.

Common symptoms often attributed to lipid deficiencies include:

- Dry skin, skin manifestations or eruptions
- Excessive hair loss in the hair brush
- Chronic stiff or sore shoulders
- Muscle tension headaches
- Problems with reproduction

Chronic Stress and Digestion

When the body is under chronic stress and has a resulting energy deficiency, it automatically reduces the production of stomach acid and peristalsis, or the muscular squeezing of the stomach to mix its contents. Further, the valve between the stomach and the duodenum is constricted so that whatever is being digested moves through the system much slower.

Stress is the most common cause of weakening of the mucosal lining of the entire digestive tract, especially in the stomach where it causes heartburn.

Because stomach acid, which stimulates bile flow, is being reduced, the bile thickens and does not flow as rapidly as it should, hampering fat digestion. This is usually enough to stimulate sugar cravings for energy. This will elevate your blood glucose level, only to have it crash as soon as the sugar is metabolized, causing you to consume more sugar and taking you another step toward metabolic syndrome and Type II diabetes.

Furthermore, when your bile is not flowing adequately, the excess cholesterol that your body normally dumps in with the bile begins to backup into the blood. Now your cholesterol level goes up, another sign that you're headed towards metabolic syndrome.

Common symptoms often attributed to biliary dysfunction include:

- Loss of appetite, especially for meat
- Frequent sour taste in the mouth
- Intolerance of fats and spicy foods
- Frequent constipation with light-colored stool

Next the flow of pancreatic enzymes is diminished, and your ability to digest lipids is further impaired.

> The whole digestive process is diminished when you're under chronic stress, and when you don't have the energy to deal with it.

This process continues all the way through the large intestine, where a restriction of the blood supply inhibits peristalsis and constricts the anal sphincter, resulting in bowel problems.

Anything to assist the body in the digestion of nutrients, such as supplemental food enzymes, could be of benefit here.

Chronic Stress and Liver Metabolism

Under chronic stress, the liver has been instructed to increase blood glucose levels. It does this by using an enzyme to convert stored glycogen and put it into the bloodstream so it is available for the brain.

The muscles also store glycogen, but they do not have the enzymes to put it into the blood, and they're using it for their own part in the "fight or flight" response. They don't share it with other organs.

We are past the point where the body cells are going to be sending their amino acids to the liver for conversion to glucose. They no longer have the amino acids to spare.

So, the liver is on its own under chronic stress. Remember, this is the major organ for detoxification in the body, and it requires a continual supply of nutrients to fulfill this purpose.

Here are a few symptoms that you may not realize can be associated with the liver:

- Frequent skin rashes or eruptions
- Excessive perspiration, or lack of perspiration
- Muscular discomfort or soreness in the lower back
- Water retention, swelling of hands and feet
- Varicose veins, hemorrhoids

Chronic Stress and the Immune System

Under chronic stress, decreased digestion reduces lipid absorption into the lymphatic system. Remember, about 70 percent of our emulsified fat is absorbed into the lymphatic system. The other 30 percent is water-soluble and can go directly to the liver. The lymphatic fluids flow when we exercise and inhale and exhale deeply.

Lymphatic stasis is not a good thing.

When you're under chronic stress, the first thing the body wants is for the spleen to destroy old blood cells. Red blood cells only live about 100 to 120 days anyway, as their lipid membranes age and become brittle, making it necessary for the body to replace them with new red blood cells, which are capable of carrying more oxygen.

How long can this go on before the bone marrow, in an effort to meet the chronic stress demand, starts sending out immature red blood cells? All this is going on while the body is also calling for more white blood cells from the bone marrow to fight off infection.

This leads to some very common symptoms:

• Anemia and other blood disorders
• Feeling fatigue, or tired most of the time
• Pale skin, lips and nails
• Low resistance (e.g., frequent colds and infections)

Is it possible for the bone marrow to become overtaxed and the immune system compromised? The bone marrow is only capable of producing so many blood cells. In the most extreme cases, it begins sending immature white blood cells, which do not function nearly as well as they do in their mature forms.

This process does not happen suddenly.

The effects of chronic stress are cumulative over a long period of time, giving us a chance to change the direction we are headed regarding our health. Our body gives us plenty of warning in the form of symptoms.

There is no need for the body to come close to this point if the stress can be reduced and if the body can be given the nutrition it needs so that the immune system and other systems can maintain homeostasis—in other words, normal function.

Chronic Stress and the Autonomic Nervous System

There are two parts to the autonomic nervous system—the sympathetic and the parasympathetic systems. The sympathetic nervous system is responsible for the "fight or flight" response to stress just described, while the parasympathetic system, sometimes referred to as the "rest and digest system," controls functions when the body is at rest, helping it to maintain homeostasis. Its function is to restore normal digestion, allow you to rest adequately, and allow you to reproduce, all of which are challenged when you are under chronic stress.

When the body is under stress, the autonomic (automatic) nervous system increases the heart rate and the force of contraction of the heart muscle; it increases the flow of blood to the body's muscles; and it reduces blood flow to other organs. It also increases respiration, relaxes the bronchi, and it increases mucus production to protect the walls of the dilated bronchi.

That describes the acute reaction to stress, which most have experienced at one time or another. This chapter is a chronic stress, where the body is forced to resort to lipids for energy, and organs and tissues have become exhausted by continual stress and lack of energy.

When the brain senses stress and stimulates the sympathetic system to go into the "fight or flight" mode, there is no guaranteed response—not if the signal is going to a cell or organ that is not getting the nutrition (in particular, specific minerals) it needs to respond. Once you become deficient in alkaline minerals—potassium, magnesium and sodium—often because of excessive sugar ingestion, you begin to develop symptoms warning you that your body is not handling the stress adequately.

Common symptoms that appear when our sympathetic response is being continually stimulated and begins to show signs of nutrient deficiency include the following:

- Problems with indigestion and constipation
- Stiff joints, especially after rest
- Becoming irritable and short-tempered
- Startle easily at sudden or unexpected sounds
- Headaches in back of the head and neck

By way of these symptoms, you should be able to tell what your deficiency is. Your body is telling you what is missing in the way of nutrition—be it protein, fat or carbohydrate, or all three—and what is needed to relieve the symptoms you are experiencing. Remember, when your body is in chronic "fight or flight" response, your deficiency has pretty much come down to fat, which the body has been forced to turn to for energy.

As your stress response system becomes exhausted and unable to respond appropriately, the symptoms change. You may experience:

- Muscle soreness and weakness
- Loose teeth or poor-fitting dentures
- Restlessness, hyper-irritability, or restless legs at night
- Lower back discomfort, weak joints or ligaments, fallen arches
- Difficulty sleeping
- Inability to concentrate, frequent daydreaming or nightmares

Chronic Stress and the Urinary System

Constriction of blood vessels to organs not needed for the "fight or flight" response reduces blood flow through the kidney, which is now unable to clean the blood adequately. Symptoms most commonly associated with this are allergies and nausea.

People think that the nausea they are experiencing is due to a problem in their stomach, because that's where they feel the nausea. But it's actually coming from the stressed kidney.

Other common symptoms attributable to the kidney are:

- Suffering from airborne allergies
- Dark circles under the eyes
- Muscular lower back discomfort

Symptoms related to the urinary bladder include a history of frequent "bladder or kidney" infections, along with:

- Frequent urination, urgency, or loss of control
- Small amounts of urine at each voiding
- Dry flaking skin, dandruff
- Discomfort or soreness in the lower abdomen or genital area

The stress reaction also relaxes the urinary bladder muscle and constricts the sphincter, making urination difficult.

Chronic Stress and the Endocrine System

Under chronic stress the body increases its hormonal secretions. This includes the pituitary gland, the thyroid gland, and the adrenal medulla and adrenal cortex, but it does not include the reproductive system.

The body's first reaction to acute stress is by way of the anterior pituitary gland, which secretes ACTH (adrenocorticotropic hormone). ACTH specifically increases production of cortisol from the adrenal cortex. Cortisol is a glucocorticoid steroid hormone, which means it has a role in glucose (energy) metabolism and is composed partially of steroids (cholesterol). It stimulates the body's response to stress and is involved with the immune system by combating inflammation.

The anterior pituitary gland also stimulates the thyroid gland during acute stress. Thyroid hormone (thyroxine) is a protein molecule. How long can the thyroid gland increase its secretions of thyroxin before it does not have enough nutrients to perform its functions normally? How many people do you know who are under stress and who have thyroid problems?

When the thyroid is still capable of responding, but becoming nutrient deficient, the following symptoms often occur:

- Fast heartbeat (e.g., feeling your heart racing)
- Swollen or uncomfortable breasts
- Moist warm skin (sweating easily)
- Neck, shoulder, arm and hand discomfort

Once the thyroid becomes exhausted, we encounter a change in symptoms. We slowly begin to develop problems related to reproduction, because lipids are being used for energy. Other symptoms may include:

- Tremors, stiffness after rest
- Dry skin, skin manifestations or eruptions
- Hair loss
- Chronic shoulder problems

The adrenal medulla is intimately related to the sympathetic nervous system. It is usually the first hormonal gland to show evidence of exhaustion. It secretes a hormone called epinephrine, better known as adrenaline. Epinephrine is a protein molecule. Symptoms related to a struggling adrenal medulla include:

- Low blood pressure and a weak pulse
- Waking after a few hours of rest and unable to return to sleep
- Frequent periods of sadness, or the inability to think clearly
- Becoming light-headed when meals are missed
- Suffering from frequent nightmares or panic attacks

Chronic Stress and the Reproductive System

I have carefully explained that when we begin using lipids as an energy source, we begin to diminish our ability to create reproductive hormones. This is because they are steroidal hormones, like cortisol. That means they are derived from cholesterol. They are secreted by three "steroid glands"—the adrenal cortex, testes and ovaries—and during pregnancy by the placenta. They are transported through the bloodstream to the cells of other organs where they carry out the regulation of a wide range of physiological functions.

You may not be aware of this, but the mechanisms and nutrients required for both males and females to produce adequate reproductive hormones are identical.

General symptoms of inadequacy for males include:

- History of prostate disorders or medication
- Frequent night urination
- Dribbling
- Loss of sexual urge
- Discomfort radiating into the groin or testes

General symptoms for females include:

- History of hysterectomy or estrogen replacement therapy
- Vaginal discharge
- Excessive menstrual flow
- Lack of menstruation, scanty flow, irregular periods
- Symptoms of PMS

The Bottom Line

If you are using lipids for energy, you are on the downhill, and it's a question of how far down you're going to go.

Your symptoms tell the story.

You go from triglycerides and blood glucose elevating, to putting on weight. You're stressing your heart, and before too long you're moving towards metabolic syndrome. The next thing down the road is going to be Type II diabetes, and after that it's drug after drug after drug.

But it doesn't have to go that far. Know what your deficiency is. Are you carbohydrate, protein or lipid deficient?

Getting the right nutrition, digesting it, and perhaps adding the support of supplemental food enzymes, and reducing your stress, can put you back on track to a healthy life.

So, what's *your* deficiency?

Epilogue

One word keeps popping up in this book. That word is energy.

As we have seen, the human body has three sources of energy—carbohydrates, protein, and lipids, in that order. Health maintenance is not about vitamin and mineral supplements, but rather our ingestion, digestion, absorption and metabolic utilization of the carbohydrates, protein and lipids to create the energy our body organs need to do their part in maintaining homeostasis and overall health.

Nowhere is this more apparent than in the case of osteoporosis, an extremely common problem, especially for women in the years after menopause, when estrogen deficiency results in a diminishing in the intestinal absorption of calcium and an increased loss of calcium from the skeleton. This has led to the belief that osteoporosis is a calcium deficiency. And yet, research has shown that calcium supplements are not an effective means of correcting this condition.

So what's going on here?

The underlying dynamic of this disease process is an imbalance between bone resorption and bone formation resulting in bone demineralization. Over time, the bones weaken and become brittle and more susceptible to fractures from what would otherwise be minor injuries, especially among the elderly. Fractures of the vertebrae, the forearm and the hip are most common. In advanced stages of the disease, even sudden movement, such as coughing, can result in fractures.

Taking a Closer Look

Bone metabolism is a two-sided coin. On one side are the osteoblasts, which are bone cells that are continually forming new bone; on the other side are osteoclasts, which are continually breaking down and removing older bone.

Drugs used to prevent osteoporosis—biphosphonates—only block osteoclastic activity. As a result, old bone accumulates and this may lead to osteonecrosis, a condition whereby bone becomes brittle faster than the body can make enough strong, new bone to replace it. Hence there is the increased risk of fracture, as well as other complications, such as jaw pain, swelling, numbness, loose teeth, gum infection, or slow healing after injury or surgery involving the gums.

Side effects of the biophosphonates include pain, diarrhea, vomiting, headaches and hypertension. Once again, drugs are designed to interrupt normal function where our ideal is to restore normal function.

Which brings us to calcium.

Calcium and vitamin D3 supplements, which have been heavily promoted, have failed to show any benefit in preventing or treating osteoporosis.

This is not the case, however, when it comes to energy deficiencies.

Which brings us again to nutrition.

During my years in practice, I was able to identify three dietary factors that contributed to the development of osteoporosis in my patients. These were carbohydrate, protein and lipids.

It wasn't just about deficiencies.

A diet high in *simple carbohydrates*—sugar, white flour, etc.— is a recipe for osteoporosis.

Bone is made up of a protein matrix which contains primarily calcium and phosphorus. In homeostasis, the calcium/phosphorus relationship should be 2-1/2 parts calcium to one part phosphorus. The processing of simple sugars requires phosphorus. An individual who consumes excessive amounts of simple carbohydrates is going to be constantly depleting phosphorus, leading to phosphorus deficiency, bone demineralization and increased risk of osteoporosis.

This is why teenagers who consume large amounts of highly sugared soft drinks experience spontaneous fractures just walking down the street. It's not the sugar that's causing it. It's the effect on the protein matrix of the bone as the body becomes phosphorus deficient.

A person will also become calcium deficient when inadequately digested complex carbohydrates disturb the calcium-phosphorus ratio in the blood, causing urinary loss of calcium.

A person can also become calcium deficient if they are not consuming or digesting enough protein. As discussed earlier, 50 percent of the calcium in the blood is bound to protein. When blood protein levels drop, calcium is excreted in the urine rather than being transported to and deposited in the bone.

The same can occur with the use of proton pump inhibitors. Shutting down stomach acid production shuts down protein digestion in the stomach which can result in protein deficiency leading to calcium deficiency and bone demineralization.

Finally, there's lipids. If you don't digest fats well, those fats will combine with calcium to form insoluble soaps, which will then be passed out of the body in the stool.

If you don't digest fats well, it doesn't matter how much calcium you take in, via the food you eat or in the form of supplements, your body won't be able to absorb it, let alone use it.

And the path to osteoporosis will be paved with lipid deficiency.

So, What's Your Deficiency?

This book has been about how your body makes energy, going from carbohydrates to protein to lipids. It doesn't matter which of these macronutrients is your problem, a deficiency in any of them is going to lead to bone demineralization and eventually to osteoporosis.

To understand this point, as the poet William Blake once put it, is to "see the world in a grain of sand."

Whatever your deficiency—be it carbohydrates, protein or lipids—the dynamic is the same, whether it is due to a failure to ingest or a failure to digest what you consume. If your body is not getting the nutrition it needs to create the energy it needs to run its systems in homeostatic harmony, you will eventually experience symptoms.

Being aware of the connection between various symptoms and the macronutrient deficiencies commonly associated with these symptoms is the means by which you can, with proper medical assistance, identify your deficiency and provide your body the nutrition it needs to restore normal function and enjoy a more healthful, symptom-free life.

Hopefully, this book has opened the door to this understanding.

Reference Charts

The following charts are for those inquiring minds that want to know more about macronutrient and micronutrient metabolism, essential compounds made from protein and essential compounds made from lipids.

Note: No attempt has been made here to write a script for those trained in physiology. They already know the process. This description is for those of you looking for a nutritional deficiency that may be the cause of your symptoms.

The Nutrient Chain

Ingestion			
Chewing and Saliva			
Water	Alkaline minerals		Enzymes
Pre-Digestion - Before Stomach Acid			
Cellulase - Amylase	Proteases		Lipases
Digestion			
Stomach Acid	Biliary Function	Pancreatic Enzymes	Jejunal Enzymes
Absorption			
CARBOHYDRATE	PROTEIN		LIPID
Mlinerals			
ALKALINE MINERALS Na+ K+ Mg	ACID MINERALS S - P - Cl		
Vitamins			
WATER SOLUBLE VITAMINS B Complex and C		FAT-SOLUBLE A - D - E - K	
Utilization			
CARBOHYDRATE	PROTEIN		LIPID
Energy	Energy		Stores Energy
	Growth & Repair		Cellular Membranes
	Homeostasis		Insulation cover for nerves
Essential Compounds			
	Insulin		Fatty Acids
	Thyroxine		Prostaglandins + Leukotrienes- Thromboxanes
	Hemoglobin		Phospholipids
	Epinephrine		Cholesterol
	Neurotransmitters Alertness & Calming		Sterols Sex Hormones
	Photoreceptors (Eye)		

Macronutrient Metabolism

Carbohydrate - Protein - Lipids

Ingestion
We usually ingest the foods we like. They smell good and taste good and we reject the ones that don't.

Chewing and Saliva
The salivary glands add water, alkaline minerals and enzymes. It is not an accident that the minerals are primarily alkaline and the major enzyme is amylase. It is all about digesting carbohydrate first, for energy.

Swallow

Pre-Digestion - Upper Stomach
The stomach wall begins to slowly stretch and the body begins to make stomach acid. This process will consume at least 45 minutes on average, longer as we age. If we consumed fresh fruits and vegetables and chewed our food well cellulase was liberated from the fibrous foods and breaks down the soluble fiber. The insoluble fiber will remain unchanged. The salivary amylase, protease, and lipase will begin modification of the foods consumed. The stomach will also add a small amount of lipase to break down lipids.

Gastric Digestion
Once sufficient stomach acid is released to activate a major protein-digesting enzyme secreted by the stomach itself, the salivary enzymes stop their activity. The food is slowly turned to liquid and drains to the bottom of the stomach.

Possible Symptoms
1. If the protective lining of the stomach is not adequate you will begin to experience a burning sensation rather quickly after the body begins to make stomach acid. This is what is mistakenly thought to be "excess stomach acid."

2. However, if the lining is strong and the blood cannot donate adequate amounts of the ingredients needed to make stomach acid you will begin to experience symptoms of inadequate stomach acid. There are many, such as gas and a sense of being bloated about an hour or so after eating.

3. You may even lose your taste for meat, or perhaps worse develop chronic bad breath and other body odors.

When Liquified Food Enters the Small Intestine

Digestion is a slow process and liquid (chyme) slowly drips out of the stomach onto the wall of the duodenum. This causes the release of two hormones that enter the blood: One stimulates the biliary system (gallbladder if you still have it) to squeeze and provide bile to breakdown fats so the pancreatic enzymes can continue the digestive process.

The other stimulates the pancreas to secrete the digestive enzymes for carbohydrates, protein, and lipids along with a watery solution (taken from the blood) to further digestion.

Biliary and Pancreatic Digestion

Whether you still have your gallbladder or not, stomach acid is needed to stimulate the flow of bile. When it is deficient the bile gets thick and sluggish and digestion, especially of fats, is retarded. Gas and bloating becomes much more obvious and normal bowel function is often affected.

Basically, the pancreas has been told what you ate and how much amylase, protease, and lipase to provide. It may not be able to provide enough enzymes for a large meal.

Digestion of Sugars

Food continues along the small intestine to its middle section where the sugars lactose (milk sugar), maltose (grains), and sucrose are digested. They have been liberated from carbohydrates by amylase and now must be further broken down. The enzymes for that are secreted by the lining of this section of the small intestine. Like the pancreas you may not be able to secrete adequate amounts compared to the amount you have ingested.

If you know you are lactose or gluten intolerant you know how uncomfortable and painful your symptoms are. The gas, bloating and diarrhea can be overwhelming.

What is not appreciated by many is that the same applies to white sugar and flour (sucrose). The difference is sucrose intolerance produces constipation instead of diarrhea. This is because the sucrose can be absorbed into the body and pulls water from the bowel with it.

Absorption

Finally, your food is ready to be absorbed so it can be used for the many purposes the body uses food for, like energy. Wouldn't you just know it, that doesn't happen automatically either. The body needs adequate amounts of minerals and good fat digestion for that to happen.

Micronutrient Metabolism

Minerals

Foods high in carbohydrate, like fruits and vegetables, provide rich sources of alkaline minerals. These are primarily sodium, potassium, and magnesium. When we consume foods high in white sugar and flour we deplete those minerals and suffer from symptoms of their deficiency. Foods high in protein and fats, like meat, eggs, and cheese are high in acid elements. These are primarily sulfur, phosphorus, and chloride. Yes, the same chloride that is used to make stomach acid.

Vitamins

What is interesting is that unlike minerals, carbohydrates and protein contain water-soluble vitamins. They are the vitamin B and vitamin C complexes, the so-called "stress vitamins." While they certainly contain fat-soluble vitamins, it is the water-soluble vitamins they need to produce essential compounds. Foods high in lipids contain fat-soluble vitamins A, D, E, and K that produce essential compounds needed to maintain health.

Utilization of Carbohydrates

Carbohydrates are used exclusively to produce energy and the body prefers them. We have already indicated how readily they can be digested and utilized.

Utilization of Proteins

The body needs protein for growth and repair of tissues. It is also vital for the control of body temperature, acid-alkaline balance, volume and transporting nutrients to the cells and carrying their waste away. Collectively these processes are known as maintaining homeostasis in the blood and the fluid around the cells. But it can also be converted to energy when needed. Obviously, you don't want that going on for long periods of time.

Utilization of Lipids

Like protein, lipids have many functions. Arguably the most important is to store Energy for use in times of energy crisis. This happens when the body will no longer sacrifice protein from its cells that should be used for growth and repair. Therefore, the body stores lipids in times of stress, regardless of what that stress is. Lipids are also important for maintaining cell membranes and insulating nerves, like the coating that protects electrical wires..

Essential Compounds Made from Protein

Hemoglobin	Found in food - requires adequate protein metabolism. Carries oxygen to cells - removes carbon dioxide to lungs.
Adrenalin	Secreted by the adrenal medulla - a fight or flight hormone. Increases blood flow to muscles, increases output of the heart, dilates pupils, and elevates blood sugar.
Thyroxine	Secreted by the thyroid gland. Thyroid hormones act on nearly every cell in the body to increase the basal metabolic rate. They regulate carbohydrate, protein, and fat metabolism.
Insulin	Secreted by the pancreas It regulates the metabolism of carbohydrates, protein and fats by promoting the absorption of glucose from the blood into fat, liver and skeletal muscle cells.
Dopamine	The alertness chemical is produced in the brain and kidneys. It functions by sending signals to other nerve cells and is influences many body functions.
Serotonin	Thought to be the calming chemical, most serotonin is secreted into the GI tract where it is used to regulate intestinal movements. A smaller portion is produced in the central nervous system where contributes to feelings of well-being and happiness.

Essential Compounds Made from Lipids

Fatty Acids	From food and require adequate fat digestion and biliary function. Have many important functions in the body.
Prostaglandins	From fatty acids, important for reproduction.
Leukotrienes	From fatty acids, important for good immune response.
Thromboxanes	From fatty acids, important for blood clotting to prevent bleeding.
Phospholipids	From food, essential for cell membranes and emulsification of fats.
Cholesterol	A sterol (lipid-like) made by all cells to maintain cell membrane integrity. The liver makes it and uses it too. It is needed to make bile, sex hormones, and vitamin D.
Sterols	Sterols act as signaling compounds in cellular communication and general metabolism. They are key components of sex hormones.
Sex Hormones	Sex hormones are sterols, and they are one influence on the motivation to engage in sexual activity.

Glossary

The following is not intended to replace a medical dictionary, but rather to assist the reader in understanding the terms as they are used within the context of this book.

A

Acute Stress: I use this term to indicate the body is responding to stress appropriately but is consuming essential nutrients in the process. If the stress continues unabated that supply will eventually become depleted. Symptoms will appear when the involved organ or tissue can no longer respond adequately.

Amino Acids: These essential compounds are the building blocks of protein. 21 are known and most can be made in the body. But 9 are essential and must be included in the diet and be made available by adequate protein digestion.

Anaphylaxis: A serious allergic response that often involves swelling, hives, lowered blood pressure and in severe cases, shock.

Amylase: A carbohydrate-digesting enzyme that is found in fresh fruits and vegetables that are high in starch. It is also made by the body and secreted by the parotid glands into saliva and by the pancreas found secreted by the pancreas into the small intestine. It converts starch into simple sugars.

Anatomy: The branch of science concerned with the structural makeup of the human body.

B

Bactericidal Effect: Kills and prevents the growth of bacteria.

Biphosphonates: A class of drugs intended to prevent the loss of bone mass and used to treat bone demineralization, such as osteoporosis.

Bronchi: Bronchi (plural for bronchus) are extensions of the windpipe that shuttle air to and from the lungs.

C

Calorie: A unit used to measure the energy value of food. Defined as the energy needed to raise the temperature of 1 kilogram of water through 1 °Centigrade.

Carbohydrate: A large group of organic (contain carbon) compounds found in foods that include fiber, starch, and simple sugars. They are the human body's preferred source of energy. In addition to carbon they contain hydrogen and oxygen, but not nitrogen which is only found in protein compounds.

Cellulase: An enzyme not made by the human body. It converts soluble fiber (but not insoluble fiber) into glucose and short chain (water-soluble) fatty acids.

Cellulose: A large carbohydrate molecule (polysaccharide) that forms vegetable fiber. The body does not make an enzyme to digest cellulose, but cellulase is contained within the raw vegetables. When the fibrous foods are chewed, the cellulase will digest the fiber in the upper part of the stomach.

Chronic Stress: Stress that has continued unabated for a considerable time as opposed to short term acute stress (defined earlier). In this book it specifically refers to symptoms that arise once the affected organs or tissues no longer have adequate nutrition to respond appropriately to maintain normal body function(s).

Coenzyme: Nonprotein compounds that combine with long chains of amino acids to make an enzyme. They are minerals, vitamins, or part of a vitamin.

Cognitive: Relates to the mental processes of perception, memory, judgment, and reasoning, as contrasted with emotional and volitional or decision-making processes.

Complex Carbohydrate: a polysaccharide (many sugar molecules), such as starch or cellulose, that usually consists of monosaccharide (individual sugar molecule) units. For example, foods such as rice or pasta are composed primarily of such polysaccharides.

D

Dietary Proteins: Proteins that are obtained from the foods we eat. We get proteins in our diet from meat, dairy products, nuts, and certain grains and beans. Proteins from meat and other animal products are complete proteins.

Digestion: the process of breaking down food into two or more substances by mechanical and enzymatic action in the alimentary canal into substances that can be used by the body. The process begins in the mouth by chewing food and continues in the stomach for 45 minutes or more before stomach acid can be produced.

Duodenum: The first part of the small intestine immediately beyond the stomach. This is where stomach acid initiates the flow of bile to break fats into small particles and the pancreatic enzymes then digest the food.

E

Edema: The medical term for swelling. Body parts swell from injury or inflammation. Protein and water leave the blood and can accumulate in a small area or even the entire body.

Energy: Defined in physics as "the capacity to perform work." Every human function requires energy. In the body energy is produced in each cell by converting nutrients delivered to it by the blood and fluids that surround each cell. The waste material produced during this process must now be removed by the same fluids.

Epidemiological: Relating to the branch of medicine which deals with the incidence, distribution, and control of diseases.

Enzyme: A substance produced by a living organism that acts as a catalyst to bring about a specific biochemical reaction. In chemistry a catalyst is defined as a substance that increases the rate of a chemical reaction without itself undergoing any permanent chemical change itself. But that is not true in the body. Enzymes are the energy that performs functions such as digestion, but they are used up in the process and must be replaced by the cells that produce them.

As nutritional supplements they can be sourced from plants or animals.

- Plant enzymes have a much wider pH range of activity, roughly 3.0 to 9.0 and can be active in the entire G.I. tract, even the stomach!

- Pancreatic or animal enzymes work in a much narrower range of activity, roughly 7.0 to 9.0 and while active in most of the body are not active in the stomach.

Enzyme Nutrition: The process of supplementing naturally occurring plant enzymes into the diet to replace those that are removed or deficient in the modern diet. Like salivary enzymes they can assist the digestive process in the stomach for 45 minutes or longer before stomach acid is even produced.

Essential Compounds: In this book essential compounds refers to those compounds the body produces from protein and lipids that are essential to maintaining health. These include insulin, thyroid hormone, adrenaline, hemoglobin, neurotransmitters, sex hormones, and many others.

F

Fatigue: Results from energy deficiency and can be brought on by physical or mental exertion, and by nutrient and enzyme (the capacity to perform work) deficiencies.

Fatty Acids: These are the basic building blocks of lipids or fat and they have many essential functions in the body. They are composed of carbon, hydrogen and oxygen, but not nitrogen found only in proteins. During digestion, the body breaks down fats into fatty acids, which can then be absorbed into the blood. Once absorbed the fatty acid molecules are usually joined together in groups of three, forming a molecule called a triglyceride.

Fats or Lipids: The term "lipid" is sometimes used as a synonym for fats. But fats are a subgroup of lipids called triglycerides. Fats are considered to be semisolid substances found in food and composed of glycerol (a sweet-tasting oil) and fatty acids (any acid derived from fat).

Fiber: Dietary fiber is found only in plant products (i.e., nuts, whole grains, legumes, fruits and vegetables) and is essential for maintaining health.

- **Soluble fiber** is "soluble" in water and it can be broken down (digested) by cellulase producing glucose and short-chain fatty acids which are water soluble. Soluble fiber has many benefits, including moderating blood glucose levels and lowering cholesterol.

- **Insoluble fiber** does not absorb or dissolve in water and cannot be digested. It promotes the movement of material through the digestive system and increases stool bulk, so it can benefit those who struggle with constipation or irregular stools.

Food: Any substance humans eat or drink for nourishment in order to maintain life and growth and repair of tissues. As opposed to a **drug** which is any substance (other than a food) that when inhaled, injected, consumed orally, absorbed via a patch on the skin, or dissolved under the tongue causes a temporary physiological or psychological change in the body.

Food or Plant Enzymes: These are enzymes that occur in all living substances including plants. They provide energy and perform all the metabolic functions required to maintain life and bring the organism to maturity. Each plant has an enzyme content equivalent to the protein, carbohydrate, and fat content of the plant. After the plant is "picked" it will begin to digest the plant itself. This can be useful in assisting digestion of raw, fresh fruits and vegetables.

Fundus: The stomach is divided academically into three sections: The **fundus** is the upper part of the stomach where pre-digestion can take place before stomach acid can be prepared. The **body or corpus** is the middle portion where stomach acid and a protein-digesting enzyme are produced. The **antrum** is the lower portion (near the intestine), where the food mixes with gastric juice and is liquified before entering the duodenum.

G

Glucose: The basic monosaccharide the body uses for energy. It is the desired end product of all carbohydrate digestion. All carbohydrates and some proteins eventually become glucose as a result of normal digestion. Stored fat is normally only used as a last resort. And when long continued causes problems.

Gluten Intolerance: A non-celiac gluten sensitivity to gliadins (protein compound with maltase) generally found in wheat and other grains.

Glycogen: This is a polysaccharide and is used to store energy in the liver and muscles for conversion to glucose when needed.

H

Homeostasis: The self-regulating process by which the body maintains temperature, acid-alkaline balance, volume of fluids used to transport nutrients and remove cellular waste, and concentration of the dissolved substances in that fluid. That includes the substances measured in blood tests such as cholesterol and many other substances not normally tested.

Hydrochloric Acid: A very strong acid formed by the combination of H+ (hydrogen) and Cl- (chloride) ions to form stomach acid. Since those acid elements must be donated by the blood it really is impossible for the body to make excess "stomach acid" since homeostasis could not be maintained. The symptoms of heartburn are caused by stress and an incompetent mucosal lining protecting the stomach wall.

Hydrogenated Sugars: This term applies to sugar substitutes such as sorbitol or mannitol in common use today. They are found in plants such as fruits and berries. The carbohydrate in these plant products is altered chemically and sold for human consumption because they contain fewer calories than white sugar (sucrose). This is only because they are not well absorbed and may even have a small laxative effect.

Hydrolysis: The process by which a substance (food) is digested. For example, an enzyme breaks a food into two parts and adds a molecule of hydrogen (H+) to one broken end, and a hydroxyl molecule (OH-) to the other broken end, thus effectively using a molecule of water to form two new and smaller compounds. Hence the word hydro (water) lysis (breaking apart).

Hypothalamus: An organ in the center of the brain that coordinates both the autonomic nervous system and endocrine (anterior pituitary gland) systems of the body to maintain homeostasis described above.

I

Iconoclastic: Attacking or ignoring cherished beliefs or institutions.

Insulin: A protein hormone that is produced by the pancreas and is used to carry glucose into the cells. Its activity is dampened as fat levels (triglycerides) in the blood rise.

Intolerance to foods: Also referred to as food hypersensitivity refers to the inability to digest certain foods without adverse effects. It is important to note that **food intolerance** is different from **food allergy**. Food allergies trigger the immune system, while food intolerance does not.

Inversely proportional: Something that is the opposite or reverse of something else. A teeter-totter if you will, one side (or element) goes up while the opposite (or other element) goes down.

J

Jejunum: The second portion of the small intestine. After food leaves the duodenum, it enters the jejunum which secretes the simple sugar digesting enzymes (disaccharidases - lactase, maltase, and sucrase).

K - L

Lactase: Lactase is a simple sugar-digesting enzyme (disaccharidase) that digests milk sugar (lactose). The gas, bloating, and diarrhea that occurs when the small intestine cannot produce enough lactase to digest the lactose contained in the excessive milk or ice cream eaten is called lactose intolerance.

Lactose: the sugar found in dairy products, especially milk and ice cream.

Lactose Intolerance: A digestive disorder caused by the inability to digest lactose, the main simple sugar in dairy products.

Lipase: A fat-digesting enzyme.

Lipids or Fats: See fats defined above.

M

Macronutrient: A substance required in relatively large amounts in the diet. Specifically, the term refers to carbohydrates, proteins, and fats. Vitamins and minerals are referred to as **micronutrients**.

Maltase: A simple sugar digesting enzyme (disaccharidase) that splits the glucose-glucose bond in maltose. Grains such as wheat and others that produce gas, bloating and diarrhea contain maltose that is bound to a protein (gliaden) that maltase cannot separate causing gluten intolerance.

Maltose: The sugar (disaccharide glucose-glucose) found in grains and flours.

Metabolic Enzymes: Enzymes produced by the body and responsible for running the essential body processes to maintain health. They are required for the growth of new cells and the maintenance of all the body's organs and tissues.

Metabolic Syndrome: Formerly known as Syndrome X, metabolic syndrome is identified as a collection of biochemical and physiological signs associated with the development of cardiovascular disease. By itself it is not considered to be a specific disease entity, but the following problems seem to be inter-related: abdominal obesity, high triglycerides, elevated blood pressure, and elevated blood glucose levels tending toward diabetes.

Metabolize: To undergo metabolism, the breaking down of carbohydrates, proteins, and fats into smaller units. In fact, the three main purposes of metabolism are:

- The conversion of food/fuel to energy to run cellular processes

- The conversion of food/fuel to building blocks for proteins, lipids, nucleic acids, and some carbohydrates

- The elimination of nitrogenous (protein-related) wastes.

Micronutrient: A substance required in relatively small amounts in the diet. Specifically, Vitamins and minerals.

Mineral: Inorganic materials found in the earth's crust. They cannot be made in the human body. They are found in small quantities in food and are essential for human function and health. The body uses alkaline minerals (sodium, potassium, and magnesium) from fruits and vegetables to balance acid elements like phosphorus and sulfur from protein-containing foods. Other minerals like iron and manganese are referred to as trace minerals.

N

Nutrition: The science of food: what is ingested, digested, absorbed transported, utilized and eliminated.

O

Osteoblast: A bone forming cell.

Osteoclast: a cell that removes old bone.

Osteonecrosis: Death of living bone.

Osteoporosis: A condition characterized by decrease in bone mass with decreased density and enlargement of bone spaces producing porosity and brittleness. Common in older women who are protein, calcium and or phosphorus deficient.

P

Palpation: It is one of four methods used in physical diagnosis to determine abnormal body functions. Palpation is the process of using one's hands (the sense of touch) to examine the body. The others being **observation or inspection** (the sense of sight and smell), **auscultation** and **percussion** (the sense of hearing).

Pancreatic Enzymes: Amylase, protease, and lipase are digestive enzymes produced in response to the need to digest foods in the duodenum. Compare to food enzymes listed above.

Parasympathetic: This is one of two divisions of the autonomic nervous system. It controls functions that assist the body in many ways to assist with rest, recuperation, and reproductive situations. This system is not involved with the responses needed during stress.

Parotid Glands: These salivary glands are located in the mouth behind the jaw and near the ear. They secrete the carbohydrate-digesting enzyme amylase along with water and minerals in response to any substances placed in the mouth.

Pepsinogen: An inactive protein digesting enzyme secreted in the chief cells of the stomach. It is converted to its active form pepsin by stomach acid which maintains an acid environment in which it can work.

Peristalsis: The involuntary (not under conscious control) constriction and relaxation of the muscles of the intestines creating wavelike movements that push the digestive contents forward.

pH: A scale used to indicate the acidity or alkalinity of a substance. The term is an acronym for potential of hydrogen. The pH is graded on a scale of 1 to 14. Acid substances have a number below 7, and alkaline substances have a number above 7. Pure water has a pH of 7.0. Blood has a pH generally around 7.4 and is considered slightly alkaline.

Physiology: A branch of biology that deals with functions and activities of life or of living matter (as organs, tissues, or cells) and of the physical and chemical phenomena involved.

Plasma Proteins: Dissolved proteins found in the blood. They are made in the liver and are not used by the cells for growth and repair. Rather they are used to maintain homeostasis. They help control temperature, can balance excess acid or alkalinity, they transport nutrients and waste, and can help detoxify foreign substances.

Pre-digestion: The process of salivary and food enzymes assisting with digestion in the upper stomach while stomach acid is being formed in the middle portion of the stomach. They work, on average, at least 45 minutes.

Protease: Protein digesting enzyme secreted in the saliva and by the pancreas. It is also found in fresh, raw protein-containing foods.

Protein: A substance found in food that contains nitrogen, carbon, oxygen and hydrogen. Proteins are composed of long chains of amino acids. Examples of protein-rich foods are meats, cheese, and eggs.

Pyloric Valve: The valve at the bottom of the stomach and opens into the small intestine (duodenum).

Q – R – S

Somatic: This word refers to the body as opposed to the mind. In this book it is also used to differentiate visceral functions from muscular or structural functions.

Stress: Any mechanical, chemical, or emotional stimulus that exhausts the normal processes of the human body resulting in energy deficiency.

Sucrase: This enzyme digests white sugar by separating glucose from fructose. It digests the sucrose found in foods such as white sugar, molasses, honey, maple syrup, or white flour.

Sublingual Glands: These glands are located under the tongue and secrete small amounts of the fat-digesting enzyme lipase.

Submandibular Glands: Located under the jaw, these salivary glands secrete the protein-digesting enzyme protease.

Symbiotic: The harmonious interaction between two different organisms living in close physical association. For example, the microorganisms (both "good and bad") living in the intestinal tract of humans.

Sympathetic: One of two divisions of the autonomic nervous system. It controls functions that assist the body in countering both acute and chronic stress. It is known as the "fight, or flight" response in emergencies.

Symptom: Any sensation experienced by a person that is indicative of a departure from normal visceral, structural, emotional, or cognitive function.

T - U

Urinalysis: A collection of tests, both chemical and physical, used to examine the contents of the urine.

V

Visceral: Relating to the internal organs.

Vitamin: Organic substances that cannot be made in the human body. They are found in small quantities in food and are essential for normal human function and health. Like minerals they are the cofactors that with long amino acid chains make up what we know as enzymes.

W – X – Y - Z

Selected Bibliography

Introduction

Loomis, Howard F., Jr. *Enzymes: The Key to Health.* Madison, WI: 21st Century Nutrition Publishing. 1999

Loomis, Howard F., Jr. *Enzymes: The Enzyme Advantage: For Health Care Providers And People Who Care About Their Health.* Madison, WI: 21st Century Nutrition Publishing. 2015.

Chapter 1

Rosenbaum, Lisa. "The march of science—The true story." *New England Journal of Medicine.* May 2017.

Cannon, Walter B. *The Mechanical Factors of Digestion.* 1911.

Howell, Edward. *Food Enzymes for Health and Longevity.* Second Edition. Lotus Press. March 1994.

Howell, Edward. *Enzyme Nutrition.* Avery Publishing Group. 1985.

Chapter 2

Abstract. *Public Health Nutr* 9(8A): 1104-1109. Dec 2006.

Sánchez-Villegas A. Mediterranean diet and risk of depression. Department of Clinical Sciences. University of Las Palmas de Gran Canaria, Las Palmas de Gran Canaria, Spain. 2013.

Chapter 3

Cannon, Walter B. *The Wisdom of the Body.* New York. W.W. Norton & Co., Inc. 1932. Bio accessed at http://www.harvardsquarelibrary.org/biographies/walter-bradford-cannon-2/.

Wulzen, Rosalind. Accessed at https://www.seleneriverpress.com/historical/anti-stiffness-factor/.

Dietary Guidelines for Americans 2015-2020. Accessed at https://health.gov/dietaryguidelines/2015/resources/2015-2020_Dietary_Guidelines.pdf/. Also accessed at https://www.choosemyplate.gov/dietary-guidelines/.

Thompson, Dennis. "Report: Sugar Industry Hid Study Evidence." *Chicago Tribune.* December 6, 2017 and November 22, 2017. Accessed at www.chicagotribune.com/lifestyle/health/sc-hlth-industry-hid-effects-of-sugar-1129-story.html/.

Goldis, Tamara. "Whole grains. The inside story," *Nutrition Action Healthletter.* May 2008.

Shroeder, Henry A. "Losses of vitamins and trace minerals resulting from processing and preservation of foods," *American Journal of Clinical Nutrition* 24. 1971.

Sapone A, Bai JC, Ciacci C, et al. Spectrum of gluten-related disorders: consensus on nomenclature and classification. BMC Med 2012 [PubMed]; *Agric Food Chem* 61(6): 1155–1159. Feb 13 2013.

Bergman, EN. "Energy contributions of volatile fatty acids from the gastrointestinal tract in various species." *Physiological Reviews* 70(2): 567-590. April 1990.

Ríos-Covián D, Ruas-Madiedo P, Margolles A, et al. "Intestinal short chain fatty acids and their link with diet and human health." *Microbiol* 17;7: 185. February 2016.

Proceedings of the National Academy of Sciences of the United States. 101(4): 1045-1050. January 27, 2004.

Xiong Y, Miyamoto N, Shibata K, et al. "Short-chain fatty acids stimulate leptin production in adipocytes through the G protein-coupled receptor GPR41." *Advances in Nutrition;* Vol. 2, 151-152. March 2011.

Theil, R. "The truth about vitamins in nutritional supplements." *International Journal of Preventive Medicine.* 221-226. March 2012. Accessed at https://www.doctorsresearch.com/articles4.html/.

Guallar, Eliseo, et al. "Enough is enough: Stop wasting money on vitamin and mineral supplements," *Annals of Internal Medicine,* December 17, 2013.

Chapter 4

Los Angeles Times. 2007 California water-drinking contest. Accessed at: articles.latimes.com/2007/jan/14/local/me-water14/.

To determine your RDA for protein, use the USDA online calculator: Accessed at https://www.nal.usda.gov/fnic/interactiveDRI/.

Bilsborough, S; Mann, N. "A review of issues of dietary protein intake in humans," *International Journal of Sport Nutrition and Exercise Metabolism,* Volume 16, Issue 2, p.129-152, April 2006.

Chapter 5

Loomis, Howard F., Jr. *The Enzyme Advantage for Women.* Madison, WI. 21st Century Nutrition Publishing. 2016.

EPILOGUE—The Last Word

Blake, William (1757-1827). "Auguries of Innocence." Poetry Foundation. Accessed at poetryfoundation.org/poets/william-blake.

Index

About the Authors

Howard F. Loomis, Jr., D.C., F.I.A.C.A., is a 1967 graduate of Logan Chiropractic College. Dr. Loomis's interest in nutritional food enzymes began when he had the privilege of working with Edward Howell, M.D., the food enzyme pioneer.

He has taught his system to professional health care practitioners since 1985. As founder and president of the Food Enzyme Institute™, he has forged a remarkable career as an educator, having conducted countless seminars in the United States, Canada, Germany, and New Zealand on the clinical identification of food enzyme deficiencies.

He has worked with enzymes for 30 years and has an extensive background in creating enzyme formulas. With his exciting approach to health and wellness, Dr. Loomis is now preparing others to take health care into the next century.

Arnold Mann has been writing about medicine for 30 years. His cover stories for *TIME* and *USA Weekend Magazine* have earned him recognition as one of the nation's leading medical journalists. Mr. Mann served as co-author of Dr. Keith Black's book, *Brain Surgeon: A Doctor's Inspiring Encounters with Mortality and Miracles* (Grand Central Publishing, 2010), which was nominated for an NAACP Image Award (Best Nonfiction Book).

Mr. Mann has also written extensively for publications of the National Institutes of Health. He served as personal writer for the Director of the National Cancer Institute, and he oversaw publication of the Institute's *Annual Progress Report to Congress*.

Made in the USA
Middletown, DE
25 May 2019